RESUSCITATION OF PATIENTS IN VENTRICULAR FIBRILLATION FROM THE PERSPECTIVE OF EMERGENCY MEDICAL SERVICES

CARDIOLOGY RESEARCH AND CLINICAL DEVELOPMENTS SERIES

Biophysical Principles
of Hemodynamics
A. N. Volobuev, V. I. Koshev.,
and E.S. Petrov
2010. ISBN: 978-1-61668-280-4

Congestive Heart Failure:
Symptoms, Causes and Treatment
Josias E. García and Victoro R.
Wright (Editors)
2010. ISBN: 978-1-60876-677-2

Resuscitation of Patients
in Ventricular Fibrillation
from the Perspective of
Emergency Medical Services
Paul W. Baker and Hugh J.M.
Grantham
2010. ISBN: 978-1-60876-668-0

Myocardial Ischemia: Causes,
Symptoms and Treatment
Dmitry Vukovic and Vladimir
Kiyan (Editors)
2010. ISBN: 978-1-60876-610-9

CARDIOLOGY RESEARCH AND CLINICAL DEVELOPMENTS SERIES

RESUSCITATION OF PATIENTS IN VENTRICULAR FIBRILLATION FROM THE PERSPECTIVE OF EMERGENCY MEDICAL SERVICES

PAUL W. BAKER

AND

HUGH J.M. GRANTHAM

Nova Science Publishers, Inc.
New York

For permission to use material from this book please contact us:
Telephone 631-231-7269; Fax 631-231-8175
Web Site: http://www.novapublishers.com

NOTICE TO THE READER

The Publisher has taken reasonable care in the preparation of this book, but makes no expressed or implied warranty of any kind and assumes no responsibility for any errors or omissions. No liability is assumed for incidental or consequential damages in connection with or arising out of information contained in this book. The Publisher shall not be liable for any special, consequential, or exemplary damages resulting, in whole or in part, from the readers' use of, or reliance upon, this material.

Independent verification should be sought for any data, advice or recommendations contained in this book. In addition, no responsibility is assumed by the publisher for any injury and/or damage to persons or property arising from any methods, products, instructions, ideas or otherwise contained in this publication.

This publication is designed to provide accurate and authoritative information with regard to the subject matter covered herein. It is sold with the clear understanding that the Publisher is not engaged in rendering legal or any other professional services. If legal or any other expert assistance is required, the services of a competent person should be sought. FROM A DECLARATION OF PARTICIPANTS JOINTLY ADOPTED BY A COMMITTEE OF THE AMERICAN BAR ASSOCIATION AND A COMMITTEE OF PUBLISHERS.

LIBRARY OF CONGRESS CATALOGING-IN-PUBLICATION DATA
Baker, Paul W.
 Resuscitation of patients in ventricular fibrillation from the perspective of emergency medical services / authors, Paul W. Baker and Hugh J.M. Grantham.
     p. ; cm.
 Includes bibliographical references and index.
 ISBN 978-1-60876-668-0 (softcover)
 1. CPR (First aid) 2. Ventricular fibrillation. I. Grantham, Hugh J.M. II. Title.
 [DNLM: 1. Cardiopulmonary Resuscitation. 2. Emergency Medical Services. 3. Heart Arrest--therapy. 4. Ventricular Fibrillation--therapy. WG 205 B168r 2009]
 RC87.9.B35 2009
 616.1'025--dc22
                        2009048921

Published by Nova Science Publishers, Inc. † New York

CONTENTS

PREFACE

Since the first use of basic life support (BLS) and defibrillation in the pre-hospital setting in Belfast in 1966, few would argue that there have been major improvements in the rate of survival for out-of-hospital cardiac arrests. Indeed, until the widespread introduction of BLS and defibrillators to emergency medical service (EMS) vehicles, an out-of-hospital cardiac arrest would mean certain death.

The initial rhythm of a patient in cardiac arrest is predictive of their chances of survival. In this regard, the rhythms with the highest rate of survival to hospital discharge are ventricular fibrillation (VF) and ventricular tachycardia (VT). In the past century we have learnt much about VF and VT, with this knowledge forming the bedrock of present day resuscitation guidelines. In the last decade there has been a truly international effort, headed by the International Liaison Committee on Resuscitation (ILCOR), aimed at reducing the mortality from cardiac arrest. This effort has resulted in the publication of the 2005 guidelines for resuscitation. While there is still much to learn, the 2005 guidelines appear to have reduced mortality from VF/VT arrests more than any before.

The concept of providing cardiopulmonary resuscitation (CPR), defibrillation, and advanced cardiac life support, in a timely fashion to reduce mortality from cardiac arrests evolved in the late 1980's. It was formalised in 1991 by Cummings as the *"Chain of Survival"*. It is the role of EMS, with regards to cardiac arrest, to provide the final critical links in the chain of survival. Aside from this vital function, EMS have been invaluable in enabling an assessment of the impact of the many changes to resuscitation protocols over the years on the mortality rate from cardiac arrest by facilitating research in the pre-hospital domain.

As VF is a more common presenting rhythm in out-of-hospital cardiac arrest and much of our knowledge of VF is relevant to VT, this chapter will focus primarily on VF cardiac arrest. It will begin by examining the birth of modern CPR and the mechanism and epidemiology of cardiac arrest and sudden cardiac death. It will then touch on the evolution of EMS, equipping them to deal with out-of-hospital cardiac arrests like never before and to make a significant contribution to research in this area. This chapter will also examine some of the issues surrounding the research that has lead to our current guidelines for VF cardiac arrests and how these guidelines have been shaped by a concerted international effort headed by ILCOR.

INTRODUCTION

Those who work in the Emergency Medical Services (EMS) are all too aware of the grief and devastation that befalls a family following the death of a loved one. For some, death is premature, occurring in apparently healthy individuals in the most unexpected of settings, such as dinner at the kitchen table with family, in the fruit and vegetable aisle at the local supermarket or while playing sport with friends. Such events remind us of our own mortality, a fact that is perhaps cemented into place by the familiarity of the context in which they occur.

Each of us has a vested interest in research into sudden cardiac death (SCD) and the management of cardiac arrest as given the right conditions, any one of us, at any time, may experience one. Dr Myron Weisfeldt highlights this fact in his recollection of a successful resuscitation he attended in 1967, where they used the newly described procedure of closed-chest cardiac massage [1]. The patient, a well-dressed gentleman, went into cardiac arrest in a lift. He happened to be the newly appointed Chairman of the Department of Medicine on his first day in that position. This chapter will begin by examining, in brief, the development of closed-chest cardiac massage and the external cardiac defibrillator, both of which form the bedrock of modern day resuscitation.

In the recent past, which can be defined as 20 to 40 years ago for most places in the developed world, a sudden cardiac arrest out-of-hospital would have meant certain death. Nowadays the overall survival rate for an out-of-hospital cardiac arrest is around 7.5%, with figures ranging from 3 to 17%. Undoubtedly, things have improved, but a rate of 7.5% is still low - especially if you are one of the 92.5% with an unsuccessful outcome. This figure is even more significant when considering the fact that under optimal conditions survival rates approaching 70% are possible for out-of-hospital cardiac arrest [2-4]. Having said this, it is important to remember, that due to the unexpected nature of cardiac arrest and the unavoidable systemic and geographic constraints there is naturally an upper limit to the maximal survival that can be attained. Some of these issues will be discussed in this chapter.

Much work has and is still being done to improve the chances of survival from a cardiac arrest. In Australia, and in most developed countries, the majority of cardiac arrests occur in the community - 86% according to the Australian Institute of Health and Welfare [5]. Accordingly, EMS play a key role in the management of out-of-hospital cardiac arrests, as well as being highly active in both initiating and participating in resuscitation research. EMS are commonly the testing ground for many of the guideline changes in resuscitation protocols that are now coordinated at an international level by the International Liaison Committee on Resuscitation (ILCOR), and in Australia at a national level by the Australian Resuscitation Council (ARC). In this chapter we will also discuss the evolution of EMS and their pivotal role in out-of-hospital cardiac arrest resuscitation, as well as their role in testing past and present resuscitation protocols and treatments, determining what has and hasn't worked. This chapter will also discuss the framework that is now in place thanks to ILCOR and the recent progress that has been made in resuscitation as well as some of the current controversies.

Finally, and most importantly, as ventricular fibrillation (VF) is the most commonly encountered cardiac rhythm on arrival of EMS crews at a cardiac arrest, and the rhythm with the highest rate of survival to hospital discharge, this chapter will give a brief account of the mechanism of VF to enable an understanding of the results of recent studies. Moreover, all of the above will be discussed with specific reference to VF cardiac arrests.

Chapter 1

A BRIEF HISTORY OF THE DEVELOPMENT OF MODERN DAY CARDIOPULMONARY RESUSCITATION AND DEFIBRILLATION

The King James version of the Holy Bible [6] contains a reference to what is widely cited as the first recorded resuscitation, circa 896 BC [7-10]. It is as follows;

> "And Gehazi passed on before them, and laid the staff upon the face of the child; but there was neither voice, nor hearing. Wherefore he went again to meet him, and told him, saying, The child is not awaked.
>
> And when Elisha was come into the house, behold, the child was dead, and laid upon his bed.
>
> And he went up, and lay upon the child, and put his mouth upon his mouth, and his eyes upon his eyes, and his hands upon his hands: and he stretched himself upon the child; and the flesh of the child waxed warm.
>
> Then he returned, and walked in the house to and fro; and went up, and stretched himself upon him: and the child sneezed seven times, and the child opened his eyes."

Since biblical times the face of resuscitation has changed markedly, with many of the significant advances occurring in the last 50 to 60 years – reviewed in [8-14]. Undoubtedly, one of the pivotal developments occurred in 1960 when Kouwenhoven, Jude and Knickerbocker, from Johns Hopkins Hospital, published a manuscript entitled "Closed-Chest Cardiac Massage" [15]. In this paper they described a technique, employed in their hospital over the preceding 10 months, which yielded an unprecedented 70% survival from cardiac arrest with good neurological recovery. This method now forms the backbone of modern cardiopulmonary resuscitation strategies. The history of the findings of the Johns Hopkins team has been reviewed at length and is discussed in brief below [16-19].

In the 1920's and 30's many electricity company linesman died from VF secondary to electrocution – it had been known since around 1850's that an electric current across the heart caused fibrillation ([20] in [21] and [22] in [10]). In 1925, in response to these deaths, the electricity companies began searching for teams suitably positioned to research solutions to this problem. In 1926, Johns Hopkins (both the School of Medicine and the School of Hygiene and Public Health) received funding from Consolidated Edison of New York for this purpose. Three other sites were also selected: Colombia University, Harvard Engineering Committee and the Rockefeller Institute.

In 1928 when the official work started at Johns Hopkins, William Kouwenhoven now aged 42, was a Professor of electrical engineering and the Dean of the Hopkins' Whiting School of Engineering. Although he had little medical experience he had a very creative mind and a keen interest in the ability of electricity to induce VF, stemming from his previous research on high-tension wire transmission of electricity.

History shows that Kouwenhoven was an excellent choice and by the mid 1930's he led the investigations in Baltimore. Based on work by Prevost and Battelli published in 1899, in the late 1920's to early 30's Kouwenhovens' team rediscovered that application of a counter-shock to an already fibrillating heart could restore a perfusing rhythm [23-25]. These finding sparked the development of the first cardiac defibrillators for application in a clinical setting. It wasn't until 1947 that Dr Claude Beck performed the first successful open-chest defibrillation of a patient with VF ([26] as reprinted in [27]). The patient was a 14 year-old boy having surgery to correct a funnel chest (pectus excavatum). On closing the patient's chest he arrested into VF. His chest was re-opened and cardiac massage was performed until termination of his VF some 45 minutes later following two defibrillations. The patient made a full neurological recovery.

The team at Johns Hopkins developed three defibrillators between 1928 and the mid 1950's [28]. The early defibrillators were open-chest defibrillators, requiring direct application of the electrodes to the heart. This was in keeping with the resuscitation techniques of the time where direct cardiac massage was used to provide cardiac output, as with the 14 year old boy above. As open-chest cardiac massage and defibrillation were impractical in the community setting, and electricity company lines men were still dying from fibrillation, there was a need to develop techniques for both external cardiac compression and closed-chest defibrillation. In 1950 Kouwenhoven began developing a closed-chest defibrillator [17]. In 1956 however, Paul Zoll, working at Harvard University, reported not only the development of an external defibrillator for use in humans but also the first successful external defibrillation of a human [28].

It was in 1958 that Guy Knickerbocker, an electrical engineer who joined Kouwenhovens team in 1954, discovered quite fortuitously that when the heavy electrodes of their external defibrillator were applied to the chest of a dog in cardiac arrest there was a transitory rise in blood pressure [17]. The technique of external cardiac compression was born. The team at Johns Hopkins spent the next year optimising this technique and incorporating the newly developed method of mouth-to-mouth ventilation. From mid 1959 to early 1960, they set about collecting clinical data on the efficacy of the combination of external cardiac compression, mouth-to-mouth ventilation and closed-chest defibrillation. Their results were published in July 1960 [15]. The combination of external cardiac compression and mouth-to-mouth ventilation as reported in the 1960 publication would later be referred to as cardiopulmonary resuscitation or CPR.

It should be recognised that the history of the findings of the Johns Hopkins team is just a small part of the development of modern day resuscitation. Their findings were based on the work of many that came before them over the preceding centuries (reviewed in depth in [8,10,14]). For example, in the late 1800's, there was experimental and clinical evidence that coronary artery obstruction caused ventricular fibrillation and SCD, and that an electric shock could terminate the fibrillation [29]. The work of Kouwenhoven et al. was chosen as they were the first to publish in the peer review literature a complete method for resuscitation, including CPR and defibrillation, and its clinical efficacy over a period of observation.

Chapter 2

CARDIOVASCULAR DISEASE AND SUDDEN CARDIAC DEATH: THE DEMOGRAPHICS AND SURVIVAL RATES OF PATIENT IN VF

Cardiovascular Disease (CVD) is a broad term encompassing a spectrum of diseases of the heart and blood vessels [30]. Of particular relevance to this discussion however, are CVD's due to coronary artery disease which manifest as myocardial ischemia and infarction, resulting in arrhythmias, heart failure and SCD.

In Australia, as in other industrialised countries, the mortality rate from CVD has been declining for many years, with some evidence that it is now beginning to plateau [31,32]. Interestingly, in countries that are becoming westernised the mortality rate for CVD is said to be increasing [33]. Despite the decline in CVD mortality in Australia, in 2006, ischemic heart disease was the leading cause of mortality, accounting for around 18% of all deaths and claiming the life of some 22,983 people [31]. Given the number of hospital admissions in the 2003 to 2004 period for patients with coronary artery disease (~ 166,000), arrhythmias (~ 63,000) and heart failure (~ 40,000) there is also a significant economic burden associated with CVD [30].

SCD, defined as "natural death from cardiac causes, heralded by abrupt loss of consciousness within 1 hour of the onset of an acute change in cardiovascular status" [34], is one of the most dramatic presentations of coronary artery disease. SCD is important to any discussion on VF, as primary arrhythmias are believed to be the cause of arrest in more than 90% of cases (see below) [35,36].

It is important to consider when reviewing data on the incidence of cardiac arrests that not all arrests are due to cardiac causes – unless specified, the data usually includes arrests due to trauma, drug overdoses, cerebrovascular accidents, respiratory failure, etc. The incidence of cardiac arrest, from all causes, is higher in-hospital than it is out-of-hospital (100 to 500 per 100,000 admission-years versus between 33 and 190 per 100,000 person-years). However the vast majority of SCD actually occur out-of-hospital [37-43]. Indeed, in Australia between 2001 and 2002, 86% of cardiac related deaths occurred out-of-hospital [5] – over 90% of SCD are attended by EMS [38,44]. The incidence of SCD in the community is reported to be in the range of 37 to 100 per 100,000 person-years (reviewed in [45]). Around 20 to 25% of these deaths are said to be the first clinical manifestation of previously silent or unrecognised coronary artery disease [46,47].

Patients in cardiac arrest are most commonly found to be in VF, asystole or pulse-less electrical activity (PEA) on arrival of EMS or hospital staff (see Table 1) [38,40,42,43,48-63]. Primary ventricular tachycardia (VT) is a relatively uncommon rhythm out-of-hospital [30], occurring more commonly in the hospital setting (1% vs. 8%) [60,64-66]. For this reason VF and VT are often grouped together in many studies. The lower occurrence of VT as an initial rhythm for out-of-hospital cardiac arrests is thought to be a function of the longer response time for EMS compared to hospital resuscitations – EMS takes on average 5 to 10 minutes from initial call to arrival on scene [43,49-51,56,67-69,70-74]. During this time VT is presumed to deteriorate into VF (discussed below). The approximate rates of VF/VT, asystole and PEA as the presenting rhythm for in-hospital compare to out-of-hospital arrests are as follows; 31 vs. 34%, 30 v. 47% and 34 vs. 19% (see Table 1). The higher rate of asystole as the first presenting rhythm for out-of-hospital cardiac arrest, again, is most likely a function of response time [69,72]. The remaining rhythms are most commonly bradyarrhythmias. The incidence of the VF as a presenting rhythm to EMS has changed with time and is now less prevalent. The explanation of this change is subject to speculation and may include changes in cardiac care in the pre-arrest stage.

Of all the rhythms that patients in out-of-hospital cardiac arrests are found to be in on arrival of the EMS, VF has the highest rate of survival to hospital discharge with an average of 19% (~ 84,000 arrests) (see Table 2) [38,40,48-51,56,58-62]. Occurrence of VF cardiac arrests in-hospital has a much higher rate of survival at an average of 39% (~38,000 arrests) (see Table 2) [53,54]. Again, in part this is most probably a reflection of the shorter response time for hospital resuscitation, including the ready availability of trained staff to provide CPR before arrival of medical emergency teams [69,72,75,76]. In studies of out-of-hospital arrests with much shorter response times [2-4], survival rates for VF arrest of up to 70% have been reported.

Table 1. Rhythm on arrival of EMS or hospital staff in out-of-hospital or in-hospital* cardiac arrest

Reference	VF	VT/VF	VT	PEA	Asystole
[38]	-	27	-	5	68
[43]	-	52	-	18	30
[50]	33.3	-	-	7.1	59.6
[60]	32	-	1	20	47
[64]	15.0	-	1.2	16.9	63.7
[65]	34.7	-	.6	24.7	38.2
[66]	46.7	-	0.5	27.4	25.4
[71]	-	23.6	-	21.8	54.6
[122]	34.2	-	-	18.1	44.6
[128]	-	33.4	-	25.4	41.2
[199]	-	37.5	-	20.3	40.0
[200]	-	36.1	-	20.9	40.8
[201]	43	-	-	18	39
[52]*	24.7	-	8.5	41.3	25.4
[53]*	-	31.4	-	37.1	24.8
[54]*	-	23	-	32	35
[202]*	-	41	-	29	30
[203]*	-	25	-	30	36

Interestingly, the value of 70% survival to hospital discharge equates well with the 67% predicted by Larsen when defibrillation, CPR and advanced life support (ALS) occur without delay [77]. It is also identical to that reported by Kouwenhoven, Jude and Knickerbocker in their landmark paper on CPR in 1960 [15]. One might assume this to be the maximal attainable survival rate, bounded by not only practical constraints but more importantly perhaps the heterogeneity of aetiologies of cardiac arrest, some of which are irreversible no matter how hard one tries.

There is great heterogeneity in survival rates for cardiac arrest as seen in Table 2. Bystander CPR and a shorter response time have been repeatedly shown to correlate with improved survival for out-of-hospital cardiac arrest [43,65,76], hence these factors are integral in the chain of survival. Consistent with this, the overall survival for all rhythms for in-hospital cardiac arrests is also greater than that observed out-of-hospital, 18% (~40,000 arrests) [38,40,42,48-51,55-62] vs. 7.5% (~ 86,000 arrests) [52-54,63].

In Australia, the pre-hospital VF presentation rate is between 7 and 16 per 100,000 person-years [43,51,60,66]. This translates roughly to between 1400 and

3400 arrests presenting in VF across Australia per year. This is consistent with the results of a large retrospective review (~ 36,000 arrests) of the peer-reviewed literature form the United States – incidence of arrest with the first rhythm observed by EMS providers being VF was 21 per 100,000 person-years [61].

Table 2. Survival for out-of-hospital or in-hospital* cardiac arrest with respect to rhythm on arrival of EMS or hospital staff

Reference	Overall	VF	VT/VF	PEA	Asystole
[38]	7.2	41.7	-	-	-
[40]	10.7	21.2	-	-	-
[42]	8	-	-	-	-
[43]	6.8	10.6	-	-	-
[48]	-	-	4.6	-	-
[49]	-	26.6	-	-	-
[50]	-	18.5	-	-	-
[51]	-	13.9	-	-	-
[55]	-	-	-	-	0.5
[56]	-	9-17	-	-	-
[57]	3.8	-	-	-	-
[58]	-	9.5	-	-	1.6
[59]	4.6	22	-	-	-
[60]	11.5	18.3	-	7.6	3.4
[61]	8.4	17.7	-	-	-
[62]	-	9	-	-	-
[62]	-	22	-	-	-
[62]	17	-	-	-	-
[62]	5	-	-	-	-
[62]	3	-	-	-	-
[62]	-	18	-	-	-
[62]	-	21	-	-	-
[65]	3.8		-	-	-
[52]*	21.9	-	-	-	-
[53]*	17.6	-	42.2	-	-
[54]*	18	36.0	-	11.2	10.6
[63]*	20	-	-	-	-

MECHANISM OF SUDDEN CARDIAC DEATH AND VENTRICULAR FIBRILLATION: THE ARRHYTHMOGENICITY OF MYOCARDIAL ISCHAEMIA

Not only do the vast majority of SCD's occur out-of-hospital but ventricular arrhythmias triggered by ischaemia are know to be the cause of many of these deaths. Any analysis of recent advances in modern day resuscitation strategies should be preceded by a discussion on factors responsible for the initiation of ventricular arrhythmias in patients with ischaemic heart disease.

In 1840 Erichsen, experimenting with the ligation of coronary arteries in dogs, established a causal relationship between myocardial ischaemia and ventricular arrhythmia, described at the time as 'a slight tremulous motion alone continuing' ([78] in [29]). It was not until 1849 however, that Hoffa and Ludwig formally described VF after induction of cardiac arrest in a dog following an electrical stimulus ([20] in [21]). In 1889, McWilliam was the first to hypothesise a causal link between atherosclerotic coronary artery disease, myocardial ischemia, ventricular fibrillation and SCD. He wrote, '...sudden syncope from plugging or obstructing some portion of the coronary system is very probably determined or ensued by the occurrence of fibrillar contractions in the ventricles. The cardiac pump is thrown out of gear, and the last of its vital energy is dissipated in a violent and prolonged turmoil of fruitless activity in the ventricular walls' ([79] in [29]).

In the majority of cases ventricular arrhythmias, such as VF, result from a complex series of interactions between metabolic and ionic factors in ischemic myocardium leading to spatial and temporal aberrations in impulse conduction [36,47,80]. Today, myocardial ischemia is known to be the precipitating factor in

75 to 80% of SCD [47] with greater than 80% of patients having significant coronary artery disease [38,45].

Premature ventricular contractions, or PVC's, originating from the margins of ischemic myocardium, have been identified as triggers of VF [47,81-84]. Indeed, they are the most common ECG anomaly preceding witnessed out-of-hospital ischemic VF arrest [81]. In 1982 Adgey et al. published the findings from 48 consecutive cases of patients with acute ischemic heart disease [81]. These patients arrested into VF, while undergoing cardiac monitoring, following arrival of the mobile coronary care team. Specifically they looked at events in the ECG preceding the initiation of VF. They report that in the majority of cases (69%) it was a PVC occurring on the T-wave of a normal beat, referred to as R-on-T, that preceded VF. The next most common (19%) was primary VT that degenerated into VF, with the least common (12%) being a late cycle ectopic beat or an idioventricular rhythm with rapid acceleration into VF [81]. Examples of these can be seen in Figure 2.

In 1989 Bayes de Luna published the results of a similar study of 157 patients with a stable health status who died from cardiac arrhythmia whilst wearing a Holter monitor [35]. Although these deaths were not due to any significant acute ischemic event such as a myocardial infarction they are still of interest as the majority of them occurred out-of-hospital and would have been attended by EMS. They found that 83% of the arrests were due to ventricular arrhythmia with the remaining 17% being due to bradyarrhythmia. Specifically, of the ventricular arrhythmias, a short run of VT with degeneration into VF was the most common (62%), followed by torsades-de-pointes (13%) and then primary VF (8%). Both of these studies highlight the role of ventricular arrhythmias as a primary cause of SCD and also demonstrate the role of PVC's in triggering VF.

Myocardial tissue is known to produce PVC's through three mechanisms, they are, triggered activity, re-entry and enhanced automaticity [85] – for reviews see [86,87]. While experimental studies have shown re-entry to be a significant factor in the initiation of many ventricular arrhythmias, they have also shown that it is solely responsible for the propagation and maintenance of VF [87,88]. This is supported by the increased risk of SCD in individuals with structural and conductive anomalies in cardiac tissue, as these anomalies provide a nidus for the initiation of re-entry (see below). In this regard, patients with cardiomyopathy, fibrosis, or myocardial scar tissue, secondary to previous infarction, are particular vulnerable [35,47,89].

Structural re-entry is enabled by a small focal abnormality in myocardial tissue providing two distinct pathways for impulse conduction.

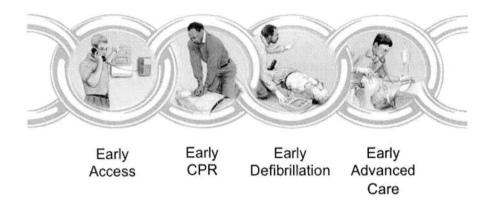

Early   Early   Early   Early
Access   CPR   Defibrillation   Advanced
                                                      Care

Figure 1. The Chain of Survival for Cardiac Arrest as described by Collins [198].

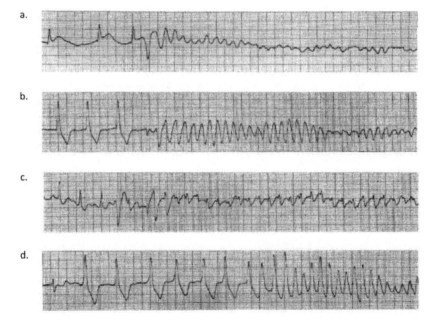

Figure 2. Initiation of ventricular fibrillation: R on T extrasystole (panel a), late cycle extrasystole (panel b), ventricular tachycardia/ventricular flutter which degenerated into ventricular fibrillation (panel c), idioventricular rhythm with rapid acceleration into ventricular fibrillation (panel d) (reproduced from [81] with permission from the British Medical Journal).

It can only occur when one of these pathways has a unidirectional conduction block and a sufficiently slow rate of retrograde conduction. Well-written, comprehensive reviews can be found elsewhere [86,87]. The conduction block can be permanent or temporary and is usually caused by either, (i) a structural anomaly in the myocardial syncytium, (ii) a derangement in the rate of depolarisation or repolarisation, due to pathology in that particular pathway, such as ischemia, or (iii) a combination of both. For example, a wave of depolarisation, originating from the sino-atial (SA) node, approaches the proximal ends of such a dual pathway, contained in the ventricular tissue (Figure 3, panel a). In one pathway (the right-hand side), the impulse meets a unidirectional block, due to ischaemia, resulting in the delayed conduction of the preceding impulse and subsequent repolarisation of this pathway [82]. The block, caused by this pathway being temporarily refractory to conduction, results in the impulse being extinguished (Figure 3, panel c). In the other pathway however, the impulse is conducted as usual (Figure 3, panel b to e). At the distal end of the pathway, the normal impulse exits and continues through the myocardial syncytium resulting in a normal beat (Figure 3, panel e). As the first pathway has now had time to repolarise it is no longer refractory, and so the normal impulse is conducted in a retrograde manner up this pathway resulting in a premature beat, or PVC (Figure 3, panels e to h) [85]. Re-entry can produce single ectopic beats, such as a PVC, or it can trigger ventricular tachycardia if the conditions are right and the impulse continues to travel in a circular motion around the dual pathway (Figure 3, cycling from panel e to j continually).

In a non-diseased, non-ischemic, structurally normal heart PVC's do not normally result in arrhythmias [88]. In the presence of structural and electrophysiological abnormalities however, the wavefront of depolarisation of a PVC, can collide with the normal wave of depolarisation propagating through the ventricles. This collision, termed a wave-wave interaction, can produce functional re-entry due to spatial heterogeneity in refractoriness in tissue surrounding the wave fronts. Such a re-entry may produce VT which can rapidly deteriorates into VF [47,90]. An example of this can be seen in the phenomena known as R-on-T (Figure 2, panel a). The wavefront of depolarisation of a PVC may also spontaneously break, referred to as wave break or wave splitting, producing two daughter wavelets that also lead to functional re-entry in a manner similar to wave-wave interaction [90].

In the setting of acute myocardial ischemia, with hypoxic myocytes and increased sympathetic tone, both re-entry and enhanced automaticity are significant contributors to the generation of PVC's [47,87,91].

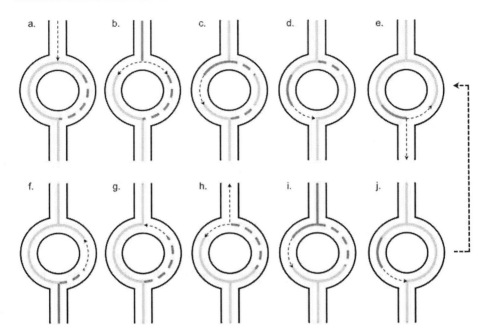

Figure 3. A simplified pictorial representation of a commonly accepted mechanism of ventricular re-entry. A wave of depolarisation approaches the proximal ends of a dual pathway in the ventricle (panel a). In the right-hand pathway, the impulse meets a temporary unidirectional block (panel b), extinguishing it (panel c). In the left-hand pathway the impulse is conducted as usual (panels b to e) resulting in a normal beat as it exits the distal end (panel e). As the unidirectional block has now had time to repolarise it is no longer refractory, and so the normal impulse is conducted in a retrograde manner up this pathway (panels e to h) resulting in a premature beat, or PVC, as it exits the proximal end of the dual pathway (panel h). Re-entry can produce a single ectopic beats, such as a PVC, or it can trigger ventricular tachycardia if the conditions are right and the impulse continues to travel in a circular motion around the dual pathway (cycling from panels e to j continually).

Automaticity is a term used to describe the intrinsic ability of myocytes to spontaneously depolarise. While most myocytes have this capability, under normal conditions only specialised myocardial cells in the conduction system function as pacemakers. The level of automaticity present in myocardial cells varies. The SA node has a higher intrinsic rate (60–100/minute) and is usually the dominant pacemaker [92]. The atrio-ventricular node has a slower rate (40-60/minute) while ventricular tissue tends to have an even slower rate (<40/minute). In times of stress increased sympathetic tone can lead to spontaneous depolarisation of normal ventricular myocytes producing PVC's. In a patient experiencing cardiac chest pain, PVC's are indicative of irritable and hypoxic ventricular myocytes, as such they should be considered a warning sign. Other factors may affect the stability of the myocardial resting membrane potential, lowering its threshold for activation, increasing myocardial automaticity and the generation of PVCs. These include acidosis, electrolyte imbalances and drugs.

Interestingly, many studies have reported circadian variation in the incidence of out-of-hospital SCD, with the highest rates being observed between 6am and midday [43,93-96]. Increases in sympathetic nervous system activity in the morning, due to postural changes and stressors, with subsequent changes in vascular tone and myocardial excitability have been hypothesised as one reason for this circadian variation [47,91,95,97,98].

The studies by Adgey and Bayes de Luna (described above) highlight the importance of ventricular arrhythmias, particularly VF, as a major cause of out-of-hospital SCD. Of course these studies refer to the rhythm at the time of collapse. As noted in the section above, the most commonly found rhythm on arrival of EMS post witnessed arrests is asystole (47%), followed by VT/VF (34%) and then PEA (19%). This difference is thought to be due to the 5 to 10 minute response time of most EMS, enabling VT/VF to degenerate into asystole [69]. Without bystander CPR before arrival of EMS, VT degenerates into course VF as the myocardium becomes more hypoxic [35], which further degenerates into fine VF and eventually asystole [69]. Effective bystander CPR has been shown to slow the rate of deterioration of VT/VF into asystole [43,64,65,69,70,75,99].

As seen above, VF is the result of chaotic uncoordinated, cyclic electrical discharge within the myocardial syncitium. As evidenced by the high rates of return of spontaneous circulation observed with implantable cardioverter-defibrillator (ICD), or in patients fortunate enough to have early manual external defibrillation, there is no doubt that for witnessed cardiac arrest with VT or VF as the first presenting rhythm, defibrillation is definitive treatment [100]. The delivery of a small electric current to the heart, a process known as defibrillation, is believed to work by depolarising a critical mass of myocardial tissue, thereby terminating the aberrant electrical activity in the ventricles and enabling a dominant pacemaker such as the SA node to re-establish coordinated control. In recent years, there has been some discussion as to whether defibrillation of a patient with an out-of-hospital VF arrest should take precedence or whether EMS personnel should provide a period of CPR before defibrillation in an effort to combat the effects of prolonged myocardial hypoxia (this is discussed below).

Chapter 4

THE MANAGEMENT OF OUT-OF-HOSPITAL CARDIAC ARREST: EVOLUTION OF EMERGENCY MEDICAL SERVICES

In the very early years following publication of the 1960 paper by Kouwenhoven, CPR and defibrillation were confined to the realms of the hospital. It was not until the mid 1960 that CPR and to a lesser extent defibrillators began to filter out into the community [101]. In January 1966 in Belfast, a revolutionary Irish cardiologist named Dr Frank Pantridge, put into practice his idea of taking the defibrillator to patients with early myocardial infarction [102]. The results of an 18-month trial of this mobile cardiac intensive care unit were published in 1967 [103]. In this time they treated 312 patients en-route to hospital and performed the first successful out-of-hospital defibrillation. In the United States, the first successful out-of-hospital defibrillation with good neurological recovery did not occur until 1969 [104]. In closing, Pantridge et al. stated, "it has been shown perhaps for the first time that the correction of cardiac arrest outside of hospital is a practical proposition."

Following the success in Belfast, the idea of bringing cardiac care to patients spread rapidly. Defibrillators started appearing on ambulances and ambulance drivers or attendants, as they were referred to at the time, began to be trained in BLS, including modern CPR [101,104]. So began a revolutionary change in the service delivery model of EMS [104]. The "load and go" mentality, where patient's received little intervention en-route to hospital, was replaced by a model in which patient's received life saving medical interventions at the scene and en-route [105]. Education of ambulance drivers, to a higher level, made it possible for them to take on a greater level of clinical responsibility with less risk to the community. It was from this increased level of training and clinical responsibility that the emergency medical technician (EMT) and paramedic were born.

In 1993 Cummins published an extensive review on the role of EMS in increasing survival from out-of-hospital cardiac arrests by improving links in the Chain of Survival [44]. He noted that while some communities had approached what was considered at the time to be a practical limit for survivability from SCD (15-20% for all rhythms and 25-30%for VF), it was clear that many communities operated with defects in their EMS chain of survival resulting in poor outcomes. In this regard, Cummins concluded that "people are more likely to survive out-of-hospital cardiac arrest when the following sequence of events occurs as rapidly as possible: recognition of early warning signs, activation of the emergency medical system, basic CPR, defibrillation, intubation, and intravenous medications." This view was consistent with the results of many studies showing that survival from VF arrest is improved through early bystander CPR [65,74,100,106-108], a rapid EMS response time, enabling early defibrillation and BLS [43,65,74,106,107,109], and the implementation of ALS [55,100,107,110-114]. Indeed, one large-scale study (1,667 arrests) has even quantified the relationship between these determinants and survival to discharge in patients with underlying heart disease, who had witnessed arrests and were found to be in VF upon arrival of EMS; Survival Rate = 67% - 2.3% per minute to CPR - 1.1% per minute to defibrillation - 2.1% per minute to ALS [77]. In the early 90's although it was clear that much progress had been made by EMS in some countries, many still had not yet achieved the optimum performance.

Although defibrillators were first used in the pre-hospital setting in the mid 1960's their widespread appearance on ambulances was a slow process, continuing through the 1970's and right up until the early 1990's in some countries [49,104,115,116] - there are many countries throughout the world where the desirable standard of a defibrillator on every ambulance has yet to be achieved. Certainly in Australia in the late 1980's to early 1990's only selected ambulances carried defibrillators, they were an expensive scant resource. The use of a defibrillator was initially seen as the preserve of a senior paramedic or a medical officer. Over time defibrillators have moved from this elite group to being standard paramedic equipment and are now considered part of the basic life support pathway. In the very early years, the lack of portability of the units impeded their widespread use out-of-hospital. Over the ensuing decades this was solved. Indeed, while the first defibrillators weighed around 90kg in the early 1950's, refinements made the next generation around 45kg in the late 50's, with the early portable versions weighing only 35kg in the mid 60's [18,101]! In the late 60's the weight was down to around 20kg with it reaching current day levels of around 10kg in the mid 70's [101,117]. Modern fully optioned manual defibrillators weigh around 5 to 10kg with automatic external defibrillators, or AEDs, weighing around 3kg. Such technological advances have made it practical for all first line emergency ambulances to be equipped with defibrillators, taking definitive care to the patient's side.

Today, all emergency ambulances in Australia are equipped with defibrillators, many having 12-lead capability, capnography and non-invasive blood pressure monitoring. One of the catalysts for the introduction of defibrillators to all ambulances in Australia occurred in October 1990. Whilst at a Polo match in Warwick Farm, Sydney, Kerry Packer, one of Australia's wealthiest men went into cardiac arrest. He was in arrests for 6 to 8 minutes before being resuscitated by paramedics. Fortunately, for Mr Packer, an ambulance, complete with defibrillator, was in the area. After recovering, Mr Packer donated millions of dollars to the New South Wales Ambulance Service, in a 1:1 deal with the government, to equip all ambulances with defibrillators [118-120]. The addition of defibrillators to every front line ambulance and single response vehicle in Australia has no doubt improved survival for cardiac arrests by strengthening the early defibrillation link in the chain of survival.

In Australia ambulance services have strengthened the early advanced care link in the chain of survival by training Paramedics in ALS. There is a degree of variation between states, but generally this includes the use of cardiac specific drugs such as adrenaline, amiodarone, lignocaine, adenosine and atropine as well as cardiac pacing and endotracheal intubation. In most states Paramedics, are referred to as Intensive Care Paramedics. The New South Wales (level 5 officers) and Victorian ambulance services (MICA officers) introduced ALS and Intensive Care Paramedics in the mid to late 1970's, other services followed. Indeed, within Australian ambulance services there is now clear evidence that attendance of an Intensive Care Paramedic at a cardiac arrest significant improves the odds of survival to hospital discharge over that seen with attendance of Paramedics alone [66,110,111]. There is a great deal of variation in terms of training, experience and equipment between paramedics across the world. This makes it difficult to interpret much of the evidence purporting to evaluate the impact of paramedics upon cardiac arrest survival. In EMS systems where physicians provide ALS (the Franco-German model), the survival rate for VF arrests is comparable to those where well-trained paramedics provide ALS (the Anglo-American model) [2,49-51,121].

Undoubtedly early defibrillation and early advanced care are two crucial elements in the chain of survival. There is little point however, in having ambulances equipped with defibrillators and manned by staff trained in ALS if they cannot respond to a cardiac arrest within a critical window [100]. Unfortunately, due to increasing demand on EMS in many communities there is a constant struggle for ambulance services to maintain response times within acceptable criteria. The current criteria are by necessity a pragmatic balance between the need for a rapid response and economic factors. Baring an ambulance on every street corner, something that is prohibited by finite health resources, there will always be a practical limit to EMS response times. This is especially true in rural and remote communities where other strategies, such as an increased reliance on dispatcher initiated bystander CPR and community AED programs for early defibrillation, may be of benefit [66]. In this regard, dispatcher initiated CPR, in both rural and remote communities, has been shown to be beneficial in increasing bystander CPR rates, which in turn increase survival [65,74,106-108,123-125].

Chapter 5

THE EVOLUTION OF ADVANCED LIFE SUPPORT

Since the advent of modern CPR and the introduction of community-based defibrillation and ALS programs, the goal has always been to improve the survival rate from cardiac arrest. In some EMS, the early implementation of resuscitation efforts was characterised by rapidly increasing survival rates. In this regard, the rate observed in the King County region of Washington State set a particularly high benchmark of around 30% [2]. From this time onwards survival rates have not risen nearly as dramatically despite significant advances in technology and our understanding of the aetiology of cardiac arrest. In some regions most of the subsequent advances in survival from out-of-hospital cardiac arrests appear to be related to the introduction of ALS to EMS [66,110,111]. Primarily, ALS involves the use of advanced airway techniques and cardiac specific pharmacology.

Starting with simple oropharyngeal airways a variety of airway devices have been used to improve airway patency and facilitate adequate ventilation. While the endotracheal tube remains the gold standard for definitive airway management, providing both a means of ventilation and a secured airway, it requires a level of skill and currency above that which is needed for other airway management techniques. According to a 2008 Cochrane review, "the efficacy of emergency intubation as currently practiced has not been rigorously studies" [126]. This review concluded that there was no strong evidence to support the use of intubation, as opposed to other airway management techniques, for acutely ill or injured patients. This is in stark contrast to the results of a more recent study from Japan, published in 2009, of 42,873 out-of-hospital cardiac arrests [127]. This study demonstrated a small but clear benefit of early intubation with regards to the neurological outcome of survivors [127]. A similar result was also found in an Australian study of 1,790 out-of-hospital arrests published in 2006. In this study endotracheal intubation was associated with a significant improvement in survival to hospital discharge [66]. Other studies, such as the OPALS study, have found no changes in survival to hospital discharge following introduction of ALS [128]. Again, the difficulty in comparing the results of such studies stems from the heterogeneity of EMS systems around the world, particularly the level of education, training and skill of the paramedics concerned. The issues include not only the success rate of intubation but also the expediency of the procedure and the judgment as to when to carry out the procedure and when not to.

Although other devices such as the laryngeal mask airway and Combi-tube have been used successfully in the management of cardiac arrest to produce an effective airway [129], there is again insufficient data regarding the effect of their use as a specific intervention on survival post cardiac arrest.

Various pharmacological interventions, such as calcium and sodium bicarbonate, have been used in the clinical setting from time to time in an attempt to improve survival. Their use, primarily based on the empirical extrapolation of their actions in non-arrested patient and laboratory animals, was common practice. They have now for the most part disappeared from practice, being brought out under only very specific circumstances. This is consistent with the 2005 ILCOR guidelines where no significant evidence was found to support their use [130].

The use of adrenaline in cardiac arrest is one pharmacological intervention that has stood the test of time, despite a lack of evidence that it significantly impacts on survival. The dose used today is still very much the same as the empirical dose first suggested [131]. If adrenaline provides any benefit, it is though to be due to its ability to cause peripheral vasoconstriction, thereby increasing central venous pressure and venous return to the heart, in turn increasing aortic root pressure and both cerebral and coronary perfusion. In the late 80's and early 90's enthusiasm for high-dose adrenaline, which in theory produced superior perfusion pressures, failed to produce a significant improvement in survival [132-137]. Other vasoconstrictors such as vasopressin (a.k.a. antidiuretic hormone or arginine vasopressin) have been considered and tried. When compared with the results from adrenaline however, the majority of studies also failed to demonstrate a significant improvement in survival (reviewed in [138]).

Various devices have been constructed and tested with the aim of improving myocardial perfusion by improving the efficiency of chest compressions with regard to rate and depth. In the early 70's a pneumatically driven piston device, powered by compressed oxygen, was described in the literature [139]. In more recent times there have been a number of pilot trials investigating a device that enables rescuers to perform "minimally invasive cardiac massage". This involves the insertion of the device, akin to a toilet plunger, into the thoracic cavity though a small incision in the chest wall. This enables direct contact with the heart and compression of the ventricles [140]. Load distributing band compression devices, which squeeze the thorax in a cyclical manner, have also been trialled. While many of these devices undoubtedly produce higher perfusion pressures and improve the choreography of compression, conclusive evidence that they improve survival is still elusive [130].

With regard to ventricular arrhythmias a myriad of anti-arrhythmics, such as lignocaine, procainamide, bretylium, magnesium sulfate and amiodarone have seen clinical use - some have maintained a place in practice, others have not. Clinically many of these agents were first used to suppress myocardial irritability in patient following infarction or who were experiencing ventricular arrhythmias but were haemodynamically stable. It was the success of some of these agents in this context that led to their use in cardiac arrest due to VT and VF [141]. For many years lignocaine has been the anti-arrhythmic of choice in this setting. In recent times however it has fallen from favour, being replaced by amiodarone. Primarily, this seems to relate to the fact that amiodarone, when compared to lignocaine, results in a higher rate of ROSC and survival to hospital admission [142]. Again however, there is a lack of significant clinical evidence that amiodarone promotes survival to hospital discharge and beyond – this is also the case for most other anti-arrhythmics [130,143].

Undoubtedly both lignocaine and amiodarone are effective in stabilising myocardial electrical activity. If however, they are successful in reverting a ventricular arrhythmia to a perfusing rhythm that is more conducive to life, it may come at the expense of a significant reduction in myocardial contractility and hence cardiac output [141,143,144]. The growing awareness of the negative impact of these anti-arrhythmics on contractility, coupled with the lack of dramatic improvements in survival to hospital discharge probably accounts for the recent change in attitude towards anti-arrhythmics in cardiac arrest. There has been a move away from the routine use of these drugs to a position where they are now used with discretion and careful consideration depending upon the circumstance.

Advances in defibrillator technology have seen changes in the wave-form of the defibrillating current from monophasic to biphasic. The evidence of their effectiveness when compared with monophasic shocks of similar energy has been one of the drivers of this change [145-148]. It is now well recognised that defibrillation causes reversible myocardial dysfunction, such as reduced contractility. This dysfunction is associated with reversible ST-segment changes on the ECG, such as elevation or depression indicative of injury and ischaemia [147]. Biphasic shocks that are effective at a lower energy appeared to be associated with less myocardial impact following a defibrillation [146,148]. Once again the extrapolation of this theory into practice, whilst making good clinical sense, does not seem to be associated with a dramatic improvement in long-term survival [149,150].

Post cardiac arrest management, which for a long time was largely supportive and expectant, has now been modified to include the benefits of hypothermia, supported by two independent studies [151,152]. These studies have been backed up at both the national and international level by guidelines recommending hypothermia for a period of time in the post arrest phase [130,153]. The evidence suggest that a period of hypothermia for 12 to 24-hours at a temperature of approximately 32 to 34° C is beneficial. Interestingly enough, although the evidence has been widely available for some time the uptake of routine hypothermia for cardiac arrest survivors has been patchy. This is possibly explained by the technical difficulties associated with achieving and maintaining hypothermia under these circumstances. The greater accessibility of angiography and angioplasty/stenting for the post arrest victim is another trend that will not only improve mortality but also impact significantly upon morbidity.

Despite the significant improvements in ALS and post resuscitation care as described above, one of the most dramatic improvement in survival rates seen in the recent decades (discussed below) appears to have been associated with the introduction of the revised ILCOR CPR guidelines in 2005 [2,51,122]. This observation supports a very fundamental line of though. That is, without the basics being done, and being done well, there is little benefit to be gained from the advanced techniques. In this regard much is to be gained from Improving both the quality and quantity of bystander CPR. Reviews of cardiac arrest victims reveal that bystanders CPR rates vary considerably from 60% in some countries [51] to around 15% in others [154]. As bystanders CPR has been shown unequivocally to be a determinant of survival, hence its place in the chain of survival, such variation is surprising. To some extent these differences can be explained by cultural differences as well as the local EMS-dispatcher protocols with regards to persuading bystanders to perform CPR. The issue of compression only CPR [155], to overcome reluctance to carry out full CPR has been studied and current phone advice guidelines support compression only CPR if the rescuer is at all reluctant to do full CPR [156]. It is important to recognise that compression only CPR should not necessarily be considered as CPR without ventilation, as if the airway is open a degree of gas exchange does occur with the changes in intrathoracic pressure. If compression only CPR is performed simple airway manoeuvre, or devices, would be advantageous.

Chapter 6

ESTABLISHMENT OF THE INTERNATIONAL LIASON COMMITTEE ON RESUSCITATION TO DEVELOP A CONCERTED INTERNATIONAL APPROACH

Historically, guidelines for the management of cardiac arrest were extrapolated from the observations of smaller observational studies and expert opinion. The field has now progressed to a stage where current guidelines are based on evidence from large-scale clinical trials, with expert opinion playing an integral part in interpreting the evidence and developing the guidelines. In the late 80's, due to the complexity of the field of resuscitation research and the many disciplines involved, the need for uniformity in the reporting of data from out-of-hospital cardiac arrests was recognised. In June 1990, a meeting was held in the Utstein Abbey, on the remote Norwegian Island of Mosteroy, for the purpose of developing a standardised data set [157]. Present at the meeting were representatives for the American Heart Association (AHA), European Resuscitation Council (ERC), Heart and Stroke Foundation of Canada (HSFC), and the Australian Resuscitation Council (ARC). It was from this meeting that the Utstein style was born [158]. It describes a standardised set of data required of any study investigating out-of-hospital cardiac arrest. It has become such an important tool that without compliance and reporting of studies in the Utstein style many journals will not consider a manuscript for publication. The Utstein style enables one to compare 'apples to apples' and evaluate the lessons learnt from different systems.

In 1996, the AHA, ERC, HSFC and ARC, in collaboration with other resuscitation committees were pivotal in the formation of an international body, termed the International Liason Committee on Resuscitation or ILCOR. The name ILCOR, or "ill cor", was a deliberate play on words referring to "sick heart" [157]. For many years, the individual resuscitation organisations had been providing a local framework for considering appropriate management recommendations for resuscitation, based mostly on empirical evidence from experts in the field. In Australia, the ARC has been in existence since the early days of modern resuscitation. With the development of ILCOR, local organisations were now working in a close international collaboration, reviewing peer reviewed literature on a regular basis and providing recommendations that were now grounded in evidence base medicine wherever possible.

In November 2005, ILCOR published it's second round of recommendations for emergency cardiac care and cardiopulmonary resuscitation [130,159-161] - it's first round came in 2000. The recommendations were the result of a critical analysis of the peer review literature containing the best available evidence at the time of review. They were adopted by all local resuscitation councils - only minor relevant local changes were made. The third iteration of this process, for release in 2010, will take into account evidence obtained since the last international recommendations were released.

There are still considerable areas of resuscitation that remained the preserve of expert opinion in the absence of a firm evidence base. Where recommendations are based purely on expert opinion, this is now clearly recognised and acknowledged by ILCOR.

Chapter 7

THE 2005 ILCOR GUIDELINES FOR RESUSCITATION: CPR BEFORE DEFIRBILLATION IN VF CARDIAC ARREST

As discussed above, in November 2005 ILCOR published its most recent recommendations for emergency cardiac care and cardiopulmonary resuscitation [130,159-161]. With regards to resuscitation of out-of-hospital VF arrests by EMS the major changes in the 2005 resuscitation guidelines, as summarised by the Australian Resuscitation Council (ARC) [162], were, (i) more emphasis on chest compression, with a compression to ventilation ratio of 30:2, compared to the earlier 15:2, (ii) a single shock for unwitnessed VF arrests, compared to the earlier stack of 3, (iii) 2 minutes of CPR post defibrillation without a rhythm or pulse check, compared to the earlier pause for a rhythm check post defibrillation and only 1 minute of CPR.

It is now apparent that the coordinated efforts of ILCOR have paid off. A handful of independent studies, published recently in the peer review literature, from Denmark, the United States and Australia, have report significant increases in the survival rate for out-of-hospital VF arrests following introduction of the 2005 guidelines [2,51,122].

When the ILCOR recommendations were published a list of controversial topics from the 2005 International Consensus Conference was identified [163]. A degree of resolution was reached in most cases, due to the availability of appropriate data. With regards to the question of whether it is best, upon arrival at a patient in VF arrest, to, (i) stop and provide an extended period of CPR before defibrillation or (ii) defibrillate immediately, controversy remained. In the 2005 Guidelines the statement made by ILCOR [164] with respect to this issue was rightly, a cautious one, 'a 1.5- to 3-minute period of CPR before attempting defibrillation may be considered in adults with out-of-hospital VF or pulseless VT and EMS response (call to arrival) intervals of 4 to 5 minutes'.

The hesitancy of ILCOR to commit either way to an extended period of CPR before the first defibrillation was due to a lack of appropriate evidence at the time. Indeed, there were 2 studies [49,50] showing a significant improvement in survival following an extended period of CPR before not just the first, but all defibrillations. Unfortunately, these studies could not be used to confirm outright the effectiveness of CPR before the first defibrillation only (see below). Especially, in light of a study, that had been published at that time, by Jacobs et al. showing no significant increase in survival following 90 seconds of CPR before the first defibrillation only [48]. The caution exercised by ILCOR in 2005 was justified when in 2008 the results of a study by Baker et al. could not demonstrate an increase in survival following 3 minutes of CPR before the first defibrillation only [51] – in fact there was a strong trend, that did not reach significance, implying that CPR before defibrillation may be detrimental to survival. The relevance of these studies in the debate over CPR before the first defibrillation is discussed below.

The idea of providing an extended period of CPR before all defibrillation in out-of-hospital VF arrest gained significant clinical momentum following the publication of a paper by Cobb et al. in 1999 [49]. In brief, this study showed an increase in the overall survival to hospital discharge of 25% following a change in resuscitation guideline from immediate defibrillation to providing 90 seconds of CPR before not just the first, but all defibrillations. The increase in overall survival was due largely to a 58% increase in survival of patients who had an EMS response time of ≥4 minutes. Although this study was not a randomised control trial, it was an observational, prospectively defined study with pre- and post-intervention analysis, yielding a result that could not be ignored. It is important to note, in light of studies by Jacobs and Baker [48,51], that there is no way of determining from the Cobb study the relative magnitude of the effect of 90 seconds of CPR before the first or subsequent defibrillations on survival. It may be that the improvement in survival was gained solely from the 90 seconds of CPR before subsequent defibrillations with no additional benefit being gained by delaying defibrillation in the first instance to provide 90 seconds of CPR.

The idea of an extended period of CPR before defibrillation gained even more momentum in 2002 when Weisfeldt and Becker hypothesised that VF cardiac arrest, if left to run its natural course, progresses through three phases. This hypothesis, referred to as the 3-phase time-sensitive model, was the culmination of 2 decades of studies into VF cardiac arrest [165]. Of particular interest was the second postulated phase, 4 to 8 minutes post-arrest, termed the circulatory phase. The hallmark of this phase is increased myocardial ischaemia and acidosis with a reduction in the likelihood of a successful resuscitation [166-169]. Attempts at defibrillation in this phase can result in refractory VF, pulse-less electrical activity (PEA) and even asystole [170,171]. The importance of this phase lies in the fact that a significant number of patient in VF arrest are reached by EMS within this window [43,49-51,56,67-74]. More importantly, evidence, predominantly from studies with laboratory animals, suggested that a period of CPR before defibrillation within this phase improved survival. The hypothesis is that CPR reverses ischaemia sufficiently to alter the dynamics of the VF waveform enabling a successful defibrillation [172-174], that is, a ROSC. In this regard, it seems reasonable to expect that an extended period of CPR by EMS, before the first defibrillation, would yield the greatest results as, (i) the average patient had been in arrest for some 6 to 10 minutes upon arrival of EMS and (ii) post defibrillation, in most arrests, there are always periods of CPR, so the expected benefit post the first defibrillation from any additional duration of CPR may be minimal.

Briefly, the first phase postulated by Weisfeldt and Becker, 0 to 4 minutes post-arrest, was termed the electrical phase. There is little doubt that immediate defibrillation is the treatment of choice during the electrical phase. This is evidenced by not only the success of ICD's, with regards to long term patient survival [175-177], but also the very high rates of survival to hospital discharge (70%) of patient experiencing VF cardiac arrest in public venues with AED's on hand and short collapse to defibrillation times [3,4]. Additionally, in patients experiencing out of hospital VF arrest and call to first shock times of around 5 minutes, the rate of success of the first, second and third defibrillations, with respect to obtaining ROSC, have been shown to be around 90, 98 and 99% respectively [178]. Whether CPR is performed or not during the electrical phase appears to have little effect on the rate of survival to hospital discharge [49,50,167,166] - the myocardium is still energy replete and benefits mostly from defibrillation. Historically it is the effectiveness of defibrillation during this phase that led to the widespread acceptance of immediate defibrillation as definitive therapy for VF arrest, irrespective of call-to-defibrillation time. The third postulated phase, 8 minutes post-arrest, has been called the metabolic phase. This phase is characterised by systemic ischemia and a very low probability of establishing a ROSC.

There is no doubt that in the studies of laboratory animals, as reported by Weisfeldt and Becker [165], an extended period of CPR before all defibrillations in the second, or circulatory, phase improves survival [179-184]. Again, from these studies however, it is not possible to determine the relative contribution of

CPR before the first or subsequent defibrillations on survival as all of these animals required more than one defibrillation to achieve ROSC. More importantly perhaps, in all of these studies VF was induced through the delivery of a small current to the right ventricular endocardium by a pacing catheter, advanced from a peripheral venous site. The results of a recent study by Niemann et al. questions the relevance of VF induced in this manner to the human condition, namely, VF arrest secondary to myocardial ischemia [185]. Specifically, they compared the ease of resuscitation from VF that had been induced through either electrical stimulation, as described for the studies above, or ischaemia brought about through balloon occlusion of the mid-left anterior descending coronary artery. In comparison to the group with electrically induced VF, those animals with ischemia induced VF required more defibrillations to achieve ROSC (9.4 vs. 2.7 defibrillation), took a longer time to achieve ROSC (7.2 vs. 2.5 minutes) and had a much lower rate of survival (40 vs. 90% survival). The authors concluded that, 'Ischemically induced ventricular fibrillation is a more clinically relevant model for the evaluation of resuscitation interventions.'

In 2003 Wik et al. published the results of a well-constructed randomised control trial, comparing, in patients with out-of-hospital VF cardiac arrest, 3 minutes of CPR before all defibrillations versus immediate defibrillation, followed by 1 minute of CPR before subsequent defibrillations [50]. This again fuelled interest in the concept of CPR before defibrillation. In contrast to the observations of Cobb [49], there was no significant difference in overall survival between the groups in the Wik study. Consistent with the observations of Cobb though, a 16%, or 5 fold, increase in survival to discharge was observed for patients with an ambulance response time of > 5 minutes who received 3 minutes of CPR before all defibrillations. Again, while this is a fantastic observation it cannot be interpreted solely as justification for the use of an extended period of CPR before the first defibrillation, especially in light of the studies by Jacobs and Baker [48,51] based on the logic discussed above. In 2004, Pepe et al. published a clinical review [186] entitled, "Reappraising the concept of immediate defibrillatory attempts for out-of-hospital ventricular fibrillation.' In this review the studies by Wik and Cobb were again used to justify CPR before the first defibrillation, following the same error in logic as others in the interpretation of the results of these studies.

The observation of Wik and Cobb [49,50], on one hand, and Baker and Jacobs [48,51] on the other, are not mutually exclusive. Rather, they are consistent with the following hypothesis; an extended period of CPR before the first defibrillation is futile, defibrillation should occur immediately, it is the extended period of CPR before subsequent defibrillations that significant improves survival. This view is supported by the remarkably similar 2-fold increases (8.8 vs. 18% [51] and 8.3 vs. 16% [122] respectively) in overall survival for VF cardiac arrests observed in Australia by Baker et al. and in Denmark by Steinmetz et al., following introduction of the 2005 ILCOR guidelines for resuscitation, with minor regional modifications. The most significant change in the new guideline was an increase in the duration of CPR following all defibrillations from 1 to 2 minutes, similar to that used by WIk and Cobb in the intervention arms of their studies. The significant increase in survival, in the group receiving 3 minutes of CPR before defibrillation, following introduction of the 2006 ARC guideline in the study by Baker [51], suggests that failure to observe any significant effect of CPR before the first defibrillation was not due to poor resuscitation efforts or techniques by the EMS personnel involved, rather, it strongly suggests that CPR before the first defibrillation is a flawed treatment regime.

It is important to recognise that part of the increase in survival, following introduction of the new guidelines, may also relates to replacement of the 3 stacked defibrillation policy with a single defibrillation strategy. The change in the compression to ventilation ratio from 15:2 to 30:2 may have also played a part. Unless specific studies are performed the extent of each of these changes to the overall increase in survival will never be known.

If the above hypothesis is correct then why should delaying defibrillation to provide CPR have little effect on survival, and may even be detrimental. Certainly, in large population studies the sooner both bystander CPR [113,168,187-189] and defibrillation [94,187-191] occur the higher the rate of survival. As mentioned previously, a study by Larsen et al. even went as far as to quantitate this relationship showing that, survival = 67% - 2.3% per minute to CPR - 1.1% per minute to defibrillation - 2.1% per minute to ALS [77]. While the rate of survival is influenced by all factors in this equation, only one of the factors, defibrillation, is a corrective treatment, having the ability to terminate fibrillation enabling a ROSC. Perhaps immediate defibrillation is simply an immutable fact of life.

Even with bystander CPR, the probability of survival still declines over time, although at a much slower rate than that seen in patients who do not receive bystander CPR [166,167]. Perhaps this is also true when the first defibrillation is delayed by professional rescuers, such as EMS, to perform CPR, in the hope of improving oxygenation and the VF waveform. Evidence for this can be seen quite clearly in the survival curves in the studies by Cobb et al. [49] (refer Figure 2) and to a lesser extend in the one by Wik et al. [50] (refer Figure 2). This may relate to the fact that while fibrillating the heart uses up at least the amount of energy of the resting heart, if not more, depleting cellular ATP stores and increasing lactate levels [192-194]. Effective CPR has only been shown to provide around 30% [195,196] of the normal cardiac output. Hence, as the duration of the arrests extends there will always be a widening deficit in the energy required by the heart to fibrillate and what can be provided by CPR. Defibrillation, if effective, terminates fibrillation and lessens myocardial energy requirements, it does however cause temporary and reversible myocardial dysfunction [197], essentially stunning the heart. The provision of 2 minutes of CPR in this post defibrillation period of stunning, as in the new guideline, provides an opportunity for the heart to rest, enabling a dominant pacemaker to gain control and some reversal of the metabolic catastrophe that has occurred. Perhaps this is why immediate defibrillation should be the treatment of choice.

Chapter 8

CONCLUSION: A LOOK TO THE FUTURE

Our understanding of the science of resuscitation has improved over the years with anecdote and opinion being replaced slowly by evidence based approaches. The future may well hold some significant advances in technology but these must be supported with system advances enabling rapid community responses and shorter delays to definitive resuscitation efforts. While technological advances can improve survival rates, the results of recent studies have highlighted that greater improvement in survival can be achieved by optimising the basics of resuscitation. Specifically, these changes have focused on the importance of reducing interruptions to CPR achieved by removing the pulse and rhythm check following defibrillation and doubling the duration of CPR from 1 to 2 minutes as well as increasing the compression to ventilation ratio from 15:2 to 30:2. It is a lesson to us all, we must never forget the basics.

Looking to the future one can envisage community CPR rates at higher level, enabled by dispatcher initiated CPR and greater community awareness of the need for timely CPR. This would be supported by perhaps a higher community availability of defibrillators and possibly a simple community airway device to ensure that compression only CPR is occurring in the presence of an open airway.

The ALS component could be driven by the analysis of the VF waveform to provide a tailored response. There may well be a variation in ideal shock characteristics in terms of waveform duration and power, dependent upon the presenting rhythm, and associated with the duration of the arrest. Similarly, vasopressor regimes may well be delivered in a more tailored format, again depending on the duration of the arrest and the presenting rhythm, all of which could be driven from the rhythm analysis software in the defibrillator.

Lastly, rapid EMS access and response would ensure early commencement of ALS, including routine cooling and greater access to angiography suites, as well as strategies to reduce the post arrest inflammatory response. Certainly, we have come far, but undoubtedly there is more to do.

REFERENCES

[1]   Weisfeldt ML, Ornato JP. Closed-chest cardiac massage: progress measured by the exceptions. *JAMA*. 2008 Oct 1;300(13):1582-4.

[2]   Becker L, Gold LS, Eisenberg M, White L, Hearne T, Rea T. Ventricular fibrillation in King County, Washington: a 30-year perspective. *Resuscitation*. 2008 Oct;79(1):22-7.

[3]   Wassertheil J, Keane G, Fisher N, Leditschke JF. Cardiac arrest outcomes at the Melbourne Cricket Ground and shrine of remembrance using a tiered response strategy-a forerunner to public access defibrillation. *Resuscitation*. 2000 Apr;44(2):97-104.

[4]   Valenzuela TD, Roe DJ, Nichol G, Clark LL, Spaite DW, Hardman RG. Outcomes of rapid defibrillation by security officers after cardiac arrest in casinos. *N. Engl. J. Med.* 2000 Oct 26;343(17):1206-9.

[5]   Australia AIoHaWatNHFo. Heart, Stroke and Vascular Diseases. Australian Facts 2004.2004 May 2004.

[6]   American Bible Society. The Holy Bible, King James Version. 2000 [07/01/2009]. URL: www.bartelby.com/108/.

[7]   Rogers MC. New developments in cardiopulmonary resuscitation. *Pediatrics*. 1983 Apr;71(4):655-8.

[8]   Eisenberg MS, Baskett P, Chamberlain D. Cardiac Arrest: The Science and Practice of Resuscitation Medicine. Second Edition ed. Paradi NA, Halperin HR, Kern KB, Wenzel V, Chamberlain DA, editors: Cambridge University Press; 2008.

[9]   Divers U. History of CPR: Fascinating insight into early attempts to resuscitate people. 2007. URL:http://www.ukdivers.net/history/cpr.htm.

[10]   Cooper JA, Cooper JD, Cooper JM. Cardiopulmonary resuscitation: history, current practice, and future direction. *Circulation*. 2006 Dec 19;114(25):2839-49.

[11] Ardagh M. A brief history of resuscitation. Journal of the New Zealand *Medical Association.* 2004;117(1193):868.

[12] Foundation AH. History of CPR: Highlights of the History of Cardiopulmonary Resuscitation (CPR). 2008. URL:http:// www.americanheart.org /presenter.jhtml?identifier=3012990.

[13] The lifesaver known as CPR - cardiopulmonary resuscitation. 1986. URL: http://findarticles.com/p/articles/mi_m1370/is_/ai_4119043.

[14] Safar P. On the history of modern resuscitation. *Crit. Care Med.* 1996 Feb;24(2 Suppl):S3-11.

[15] Kouwenhoven WB, Jude JR, Knickerbocker GG. Closed-chest cardiac massage. *JAMA.* 1960 Jul 9;173:1064-7.

[16] Cavagnaro L, Kiviat BJ. Simply CPR. Johns Hopkins School of Medicine. 2000. URL: http://www.jhu.edu/~jhumag/0400web/12.html.

[17] Acosta P, Varon J, Sternbach GL, Baskett P. Resuscitation great. Kouwenhoven, Jude and Knickerbocker: The introduction of defibrillation and external chest compressions into modern resuscitation. Resuscitation. 2005 Feb;64(2):139-43.

[18] Worthington J. The engineer who could. Baltimore: Johns Hopkins School of Medicine. 1998. URL:http://www. hopkinsmedicine. org/hmn/W98/engr.html.

[19] Fye WB. Ventricular fibrillation and defibrillation: historical perspectives with emphasis on the contributions of John MacWilliam, Carl Wiggers, and William Kouwenhoven. *Circulation.* 1985;71:858-65.

[20] Hoffa M, Ludwig C. Einige neue Versuche uber Herzbewegung. Zeitschrift Rationelle Medizin. 1850;9:107-44.

[21] Efimov IR. History of fibrillation and defibrillation. 2004. URL:http:// efimov.wustl.edu/defibrillation/history/defibrillation_history.htm.

[22] Hoffa M, Ludwig C. Einige neue versuche uber herzbewegung. . Zeitschrift Rationelle Medizin 1850;9:107-44.

[23] Hooker DR. On the recovery of the heart in electric shock. *American Journal of Physiology.* 1929;91:305-28.

[24] Hooker DR, Kouwenhoven WB, Langworthy O. The effect of alternating electric current on the heart. *American Journal of Physiology.* 1933;103:444-54.

[25] Kouwenhoven WB, Hooker DR. Resuscitation by countershock. Electrical Engineering. 1933;52:475-7.

[26] Beck CS, Pritchard WH, Feil HS. Ventricular fibrillation of long duration abolished by electric shock. *JAMA.* 1947 December 13;135(15):985-6.

[27] Moss AJ. History of Electrocardiology. Ann Noninvasive Electrocardiol. 1998 July;3(3):281-3.

[28] Romanowski P. External defibrillator. 2007. URL:http:// www.madehow.com /Volume-7/External-Defibrillator.html.

[29] Janse MJ. A brief history of sudden cardiac death and its therapy. *Pharmacol. Ther.* 2003 Oct;100(1):89-99.

[30] Cardiovascular Disease in Australia: A Snapshot, 2004-05. Australian Bureau of Statistics. 2006. URL:http://www.abs.gov.au /ausstats /abs@.nsf/mf/4821.0.55.001.

[31] Causes of Death, Australia, 2006. Australian Bureau of Statistics. 2006. URL:http://www.abs.gov.au/ausstats/abs@.nsf/mf/3303.0.

[32] Wilson A, Siskind V. Coronary heart disease mortality in Australia: is mortality starting to increase among young men? *Int. J. Epidemiol.* 1995 Aug;24(4):678-84.

[33] Epstein FH. Recent international changes in coronary heart disease mortality. *Nutr. Metab.* 1980;24 Suppl 1:45-9.

[34] Myerburg RJ, Castellanos A. Chapter 36. Cardiac Arrest and Sudden Cardiac Death. In: Libby P, Bonow RO, Mann DL, Zipes DP, editors. Libby: Braunwald's Heart Disease: A Textbook of Cardiovascular Medicine. Philadelphia: *Saunders Elsevier;* 2008. p. 933-71.

[35] Bayes de Luna A, Coumel P, Leclercq JF. Ambulatory sudden cardiac death: mechanisms of production of fatal arrhythmia on the basis of data from 157 cases. *Am. Heart J.* 1989 Jan;117(1):151-9.

[36] Martinez-Rubio A, Bayes-Genis A, Guindo J, Bayes de Luna A. Sudden cardiac death. *Contributions to Science.* 1999;1(2):147-57.

[37] Foundation AH. Out-of-Hospital Cardiac Arrest. Statistical Fact Sheet. 2008 Update. In: Foundation AH, editor.: *American Heart Foundation*; 2008. p. 3.

[38] Moore MJ, Glover BM, McCann CJ, Cromie NA, Ferguson P, Catney DC, et al. Demographic and temporal trends in out of hospital sudden cardiac death in Belfast. *Heart.* 2006 Mar;92(3):311-5.

[39] Yasuyuki H, Atsushi H, Hiroshi M, Hirotsugu A, Isao N, Hitoshi Y. Incidence and Characteristics of Out-of-Hospital Cardiac Arrest in 5 International Regions. A Comparison of Prospective Studies. *Journal of Japanese Association for Acute Medicine.* 2000;11(1):8-15.

[40] Atwood C, Eisenberg MS, Herlitz J, Rea TD. Incidence of EMS-treated out-of-hospital cardiac arrest in Europe. *Resuscitation.* 2005 Oct;67(1):75-80.

[41] Capewell S, O'Flaherty M. What explains declining coronary mortality? Lessons and warnings. *Heart.* 2008 Sep;94(9):1105-8.

[42] Chugh SS, Jui J, Gunson K, Stecker EC, John BT, Thompson B, et al. Current burden of sudden cardiac death: multiple source surveillance versus retrospective death certificate-based review in a large U.S. community. *J. Am. Coll Cardiol.* 2004 Sep 15;44(6):1268-75.

[43] Finn JC, Jacobs IG, Holman CD, Oxer HF. Outcomes of out-of-hospital cardiac arrest patients in Perth, Western Australia, 1996-1999. *Resuscitation.* 2001 Dec;51(3):247-55.

[44] Cummins RO. Emergency medical services and sudden cardiac arrest: the "chain of survival" concept. *Annu. Rev. Public Health.* 1993;14:313-33.

[45] Chugh SS, Reinier K, Teodorescu C, Evanado A, Kehr E, Al Samara M, et al. Epidemiology of sudden cardiac death: clinical and research implications. *Prog. Cardiovasc. Dis.* 2008 Nov-Dec;51(3):213-28.

[46] Myerburg RJ, Kessler KM, Castellanos A. Sudden cardiac death: epidemiology, transient risk, and intervention assessment. *Ann. Intern. Med.* 1993 Dec 15;119(12):1187-97.

[47] Luqman N, Sung RJ, Wang CL, Kuo CT. Myocardial ischemia and ventricular fibrillation: pathophysiology and clinical implications. *Int. J. Cardiol.* 2007 Jul 31;119(3):283-90.

[48] Jacobs IG, Finn JC, Oxer HF, Jelinek GA. CPR before defibrillation in out-of-hospital cardiac arrest: a randomized trial. *Emerg. Med. Australas.* 2005 Feb;17(1):39-45.

[49] Cobb LA, Fahrenbruch CE, Walsh TR, Copass MK, Olsufka M, Breskin M, et al. Influence of cardiopulmonary resuscitation prior to defibrillation in patients with out-of-hospital ventricular fibrillation. *JAMA.* 1999 Apr 7;281(13):1182-8.

[50] Wik L, Hansen TB, Fylling F, Steen T, Vaagenes P, Auestad BH, et al. Delaying defibrillation to give basic cardiopulmonary resuscitation to patients with out-of-hospital ventricular fibrillation: a randomized trial. *JAMA.* 2003 Mar 19;289(11):1389-95.

[51] Baker PW, Conway J, Cotton C, Ashby DT, Smyth J, Woodman RJ, et al. Defibrillation or cardiopulmonary resuscitation first for patients with out-of-hospital cardiac arrests found by paramedics to be in ventricular fibrillation? A randomised control trial. *Resuscitation.* 2008 Dec;79(3):424-31.

[52] Cooper S, Cade J. Predicting survival, in-hospital cardiac arrests: resuscitation survival variables and training effectiveness. *Resuscitation.* 1997 Aug;35(1):17-22.

[53] Gwinnutt CL, Columb M, Harris R. Outcome after cardiac arrest in adults in UK hospitals: effect of the 1997 guidelines. *Resuscitation.* 2000 Oct;47(2):125-35.

[54] Nadkarni VM, Larkin GL, Peberdy MA, Carey SM, Kaye W, Mancini ME, et al. First documented rhythm and clinical outcome from in-hospital cardiac arrest among children and adults. *JAMA.* 2006 Jan 4;295(1):50-7.

[55] Vayrynen T, Kuisma M, Maatta T, Boyd J. Medical futility in asystolic out-of-hospital cardiac arrest. *Acta Anaesthesiol. Scand.* 2008 Jan;52(1):81-7.

[56] Myerburg RJ, Fenster J, Velez M, Rosenberg D, Lai S, Kurlansky P, et al. Impact of community-wide police car deployment of automated external defibrillators on survival from out-of-hospital cardiac arrest. *Circulation.* 2002 Aug 27;106(9):1058-64.

[57] Byrne R, Constant O, Smyth Y, Callagy G, Nash P, Daly K, et al. Multiple source surveillance incidence and aetiology of out-of-hospital sudden cardiac death in a rural population in the West of Ireland. *Eur. Heart J.* 2008 Jun;29(11):1418-23.

[58] Holmberg M, Holmberg S, Herlitz J. Incidence, duration and survival of ventricular fibrillation in out-of-hospital cardiac arrest patients in sweden. *Resuscitation.* 2000 Mar;44(1):7-17.

[59] Nichol G, Thomas E, Callaway CW, Hedges J, Powell JL, Aufderheide TP, et al. Regional variation in out-of-hospital cardiac arrest incidence and outcome. *JAMA.* 2008 Sep 24;300(12):1423-31.

[60] Cheung W, Flynn M, Thanakrishnan G, Milliss DM, Fugaccia E. Survival after out-of-hospital cardiac arrest in Sydney, Australia. *Crit. Care Resusc.* 2006 Dec;8(4):321-7.

[61] Rea TD, Eisenberg MS, Sinibaldi G, White RD. Incidence of EMS-treated out-of-hospital cardiac arrest in the United States. *Resuscitation.* 2004 Oct;63(1):17-24.

[62] McR. Meyer AD, Cameron PA, Smith KL, McNeil JJ. Out-of-hospital cardiac arrest. *Med. J. Aust.* 2000 Jan 17;172(2):73-6.

[63] de Vos R, de Haes HC, Koster RW, de Haan RJ. Quality of survival after cardiopulmonary resuscitation. *Arch. Intern. Med.* 1999 Feb 8;159(3):249-54.

[64] SOS-KANTO. Incidence of ventricular fibrillation in patients with out-of-hospital cardiac arrest in Japan: survey of survivors after out-of-hospital cardiac arrest in Kanto area (SOS-KANTO). *Circ. J.* 2005 Oct;69(10):1157-62.

[65] Fridman M, Barnes V, Whyman A, Currell A, Bernard S, Walker T, et al. A model of survival following pre-hospital cardiac arrest based on the Victorian Ambulance Cardiac Arrest Register. *Resuscitation.* 2007 Nov;75(2):311-22.

[66] Jennings PA, Cameron P, Walker T, Bernard S, Smith K. Out-of-hospital cardiac arrest in Victoria: rural and urban outcomes. *Med J. Aust.* 2006 Aug 7;185(3):135-9.

[67] Callaham M, Madsen CD. Relationship of timeliness of paramedic advanced life support interventions to outcome in out-of-hospital cardiac arrest treated by first responders with defibrillators. *Ann. Emerg. Med.* 1996 May;27(5):638-48.

[68] De Maio VJ, Stiell IG, Wells GA, Spaite DW. Cardiac arrest witnessed by emergency medical services personnel: descriptive epidemiology, prodromal symptoms, and predictors of survival. OPALS study group. *Ann. Emerg. Med.* 2000 Feb;35(2):138-46.

[69] Waalewijn RA, Nijpels MA, Tijssen JG, Koster RW. Prevention of deterioration of ventricular fibrillation by basic life support during out-of-hospital cardiac arrest. *Resuscitation.* 2002 Jul;54(1):31-6.

[70] Dowie R, Campbell H, Donohoe R, Clarke P. 'Event tree' analysis of out-of-hospital cardiac arrest data: confirming the importance of bystander CPR. *Resuscitation.* 2003 Feb;56(2):173-81.

[71] Polentini MS, Pirrallo RG, McGill W. The changing incidence of ventricular fibrillation in Milwaukee, Wisconsin (1992-2002). *Prehosp. Emerg. Care.* 2006 Jan-Mar;10(1):52-60.

[72] Pell JP, Sirel JM, Marsden AK, Ford I, Cobbe SM. Effect of reducing ambulance response times on deaths from out of hospital cardiac arrest: cohort study. *BMJ.* 2001 Jun 9;322(7299):1385-8.

[73] Fredriksson M, Herlitz J, Engdahl J. Nineteen years' experience of out-of-hospital cardiac arrest in Gothenburg--reported in Utstein style. *Resuscitation.* 2003 Jul;58(1):37-47.

[74] Stiell IG, Wells GA, DeMaio VJ, Spaite DW, Field BJ, 3rd, Munkley DP, et al. Modifiable factors associated with improved cardiac arrest survival in a multicenter basic life support/defibrillation system: OPALS Study Phase I results. Ontario Prehospital Advanced Life Support. *Ann. Emerg. Med.* 1999 Jan;33(1):44-50.

[75] Swor RA, Boji B, Cynar M, Sadler E, Basse E, Dalbec DL, et al. Bystander vs EMS first-responder CPR: initial rhythm and outcome in witnessed nonmonitored out-of-hospital cardiac arrest. *Acad. Emerg. Med.* 1995 Jun;2(6):494-8.

[76] Swor RA, Jackson RE, Cynar M, Sadler E, Basse E, Boji B, et al. Bystander CPR, ventricular fibrillation, and survival in witnessed, unmonitored out-of-hospital cardiac arrest. *Ann. Emerg. Med.* 1995 Jun;25(6):780-4.

[77] Larsen MP, Eisenberg MS, Cummins RO, Hallstrom AP. Predicting survival from out-of-hospital cardiac arrest: a graphic model. *Ann. Emerg. Med.* 1993 Nov;22(11):1652-8.

[78] Erichsen JE. On the influence of the coronary circulation on the action of the heart. *Lond Med. Gaz.* 1841-1842;2:561-5.

[79] McWilliam JA. Cardiac failure and sudden death. Br Med J. 1989;1:6-7.

[80] Cascio WE. Myocardial ischemia: what factors determine arrhythmogenesis? *J. Cardiovasc. Electrophysiol.* 2001 Jun;12(6):726-9.

[81] Adgey AA, Devlin JE, Webb SW, Mulholland HC. Initiation of ventricular fibrillation outside hospital in patients with acute ischaemic heart disease. *Br. Heart J.* 1982 Jan;47(1):55-61.

[82] De Groot JR, Coronel R. Acute ischemia-induced gap junctional uncoupling and arrhythmogenesis. *Cardiovasc. Res.* 2004 May 1;62(2):323-34.

[83] Enjoji Y, Mizobuchi M, Shibata K, Yokouchi I, Funatsu A, Kanbayashi D, et al. Catheter ablation for an incessant form of antiarrhythmic drug-resistant ventricular fibrillation after acute coronary syndrome. *Pacing Clin. Electrophysiol.* 2006 Jan;29(1):102-5.

[84] Varma N. Onset of ventricular fibrillation: opportunities for paced prevention. *Pacing Clin. Electrophysiol.* 2008 Feb;31(2):141-3.

[85] Keany JE, Desai AD. Premature Ventricular Contraction. e-Medicine. 2008. URL:http://emedicine.medscape.com/article/761148-overview.

[86] Grant AO, Durrani S. Chapter 57. Mechanisms of Cardiac Arrhythmias. In: Topol EJ, editor. Textbook of Cardiovascular Medicine. 3rd ed. Philadelphia: Lippincott Williams and Wilkins; 2007.

[87] Rubart M, Zipes DP. Chapter 31 - Genesis of Cardiac Arrhythmias: Electrophysiological Considerations. In: Libby P, Bonow RO, Mann DL, Zipes DP, editors. Libby: Braunwald's Heart Disease: A Textbook of Cardiovascular Medicine. Philadelphia: *Sanders Elsevier*; 2008. p. 727-61.

[88] Rho RW, Page RL. Chapter 39. Ventricular Arrhythmias. In: Fuster V, Walsh R, O'Rourke RA, Poole-Wilson P, editors. Hurst's the Heart. 12th ed. New York: McGraw Hill Medical; 2008.

[89] Okada T, Yamada T, Murakami Y, Yoshida N, Ninomiya Y, Toyama J. Mapping and ablation of trigger premature ventricular contractions in a case of electrical storm associated with ischemic cardiomyopathy. *Pacing Clin. Electrophysiol.* 2007 Mar;30(3):440-3.

[90] Kim YH, Yashima M, Wu TJ, Doshi R, Chen PS, Karagueuzian HS. Mechanism of procainamide-induced prevention of spontaneous wave break during ventricular fibrillation. Insight into the maintenance of fibrillation wave fronts. *Circulation.* 1999 Aug 10;100(6):666-74.

[91] Ulucan C, Cetintas V, Tetik A, Eroglu Z, Kayikcioglu M, Can LH, et al. Beta1 and beta2-adrenergic receptor polymorphisms and idiopathic ventricular arrhythmias. *J. Cardiovasc. Electrophysiol.* 2008 Oct; 19(10):1053-8.

[92] Huszar RJ. Basic Dysrhythmias. Allen A, editor. St Louis: Mosby; 2002.

[93] Jones-Crawford JL, Parish DC, Smith BE, Dane FC. Resuscitation in the hospital: circadian variation of cardiopulmonary arrest. *Am. J. Med.* 2007 Feb;120(2):158-64.

[94] Martens PR, Calle P, Van den Poel B, Lewi P. Further prospective evidence of a circadian variation in the frequency of call for sudden cardiac death. Belgian Cardiopulmonary Cerebral Resuscitation Study Group. *Intensive Care Med.* 1995 Jan;21(1):45-9.

[95] Lateef F, Ong ME, Alfred T, Leong BS, Ong VY, Tiah L, et al. Circadian rhythm in cardiac arrest: the Singapore experience. *Singapore Med. J.* 2008 Sep;49(9):719-23.

[96] Savopoulos C, Ziakas A, Hatzitolios A, Delivoria C, Kounanis A, Mylonas S, et al. Circadian rhythm in sudden cardiac death: a retrospective study of 2,665 cases. *Angiology.* 2006 Mar-Apr;57(2):197-204.

[97] Samuels MA. The brain-heart connection. *Circulation.* 2007 Jul 3;116(1):77-84.

[98] Lerman BB, Stein K, Engelstein ED, Battleman DS, Lippman N, Bei D, et al. Mechanism of repetitive monomorphic ventricular tachycardia. *Circulation.* 1995 Aug 1;92(3):421-9.

[99] Tovar OH, Jones JL. Electrophysiological deterioration during long-duration ventricular fibrillation. *Circulation.* 2000 Dec 5;102(23):2886-91.

[100] Valenzuela TD, Roe DJ, Cretin S, Spaite DW, Larsen MP. Estimating effectiveness of cardiac arrest interventions: a logistic regression survival model. *Circulation.* 1997 Nov 18;96(10):3308-13.

[101] Beonadonna P. The History of Paramedics. Rochester, New York: Public Safety Training Centre, Monroe Community College. 2003. URL:http://www.monroecc.edu/depts/pstc/backup/parashis.htm.

[102] Shurlock B. Pioneers in cardiology: Frank Pantridge,CBE, MC, MD, FRCP, FACC. *Circulation.* 2007 Dec 18;116(25):f145-8.

[103] Pantridge JF, Geddes JS. A mobile intensive-care unit in the management of myocardial infarction. Lancet. 1967 Aug 5;2(7510):271-3.

[104] A little history. URL:http://www.angelfire.com /co/ fantasyfigures /710history.html.

[105] Ambulance. Wikipedia. 2008. URL:http://en.wikipedia.org /wiki /Ambulance.

[106] Herlitz J, Svensson L, Engdahl J, Silfverstolpe J. Characteristics and outcome in out-of-hospital cardiac arrest when patients are found in a non-shockable rhythm. *Resuscitation.* 2008 Jan;76(1):31-6.

[107] Nichol G, Stiell IG, Laupacis A, Pham B, De Maio VJ, Wells GA. A cumulative meta-analysis of the effectiveness of defibrillator-capable emergency medical services for victims of out-of-hospital cardiac arrest. *Ann. Emerg. Med.* 1999 Oct;34(4 Pt 1):517-25.

[108] Spaite DW, Hanlon T, Criss EA, Valenzuela TD, Wright AL, Keeley KT, et al. Prehospital cardiac arrest: the impact of witnessed collapse and bystander CPR in a metropolitan EMS system with short response times. *Ann. Emerg. Med.* 1990 Nov;19(11):1264-9.

[109] Estner HL, Gunzel C, Ndrepepa G, William F, Blaumeiser D, Rupprecht B, et al. Outcome after out-of-hospital cardiac arrest in a physician-staffed emergency medical system according to the Utstein style. *Am. Heart J.* 2007 May;153(5):792-9.

[110] Woodall J, McCarthy M, Johnston T, Tippett V, Bonham R. Impact of advanced cardiac life support-skilled paramedics on survival from out-of-hospital cardiac arrest in a statewide emergency medical service. *Emerg. Med. J.* 2007 Feb;24(2):134-8.

[111] Grantham HJ. *New Paradigm. paramedic.* 1997.

[112] Kette F, Pellis T. Increased survival despite a reduction in out-of-hospital ventricular fibrillation in north-east Italy. *Resuscitation.* 2007 Jan;72(1):52-8.

[113] Weston CF, Wilson RJ, Jones SD. Predicting survival from out-of-hospital cardiac arrest: a multivariate analysis. *Resuscitation.* 1997 Feb;34(1):27-34.

[114] Dickinson ET, Schneider RM, Verdile VP. The impact of prehospital physicians on out-of-hospital nonasystolic cardiac arrest. *Prehosp. Emerg. Care.* 1997 Jul-Sep;1(3):132-5.

[115] Early Defibrillation. Rochester Police EMS History. 2007. URL:http://www.rochestermn.gov/departments/police/defibrillation/EDP%20History.asp.

[116] Scott IA, Fitzgerald GJ. Early defibrillation in out-of-hospital sudden cardiac death: an Australian experience. *Arch. Emerg. Med.* 1993 Mar;10(1):1-7.

[117] Physio-Control International Corp. History of Life-Pak and other commercial defibrillators. 1997. URL:http://www. fundinguniverse. com/company-histories/PhysioControl-International-Corp-Company-History.html.

[118] Davies   O.   Defibrillation.   Wikipedia.   2008.   URL:http://en. wikipedia.org/wiki /User:Owain.davies/Defibrillation.

[119] Kerry   Packer.   Wikipedia.   2009.   URL:http://en.wikipedia.org /wiki/Kerry_Packer.

[120] Obituary: Kerry Packer. The Times On-line. 2005. URL:http: //www.timesonline.co.uk/tol/comment/obituaries/article782808.ece.

[121] Fleischmann T, Fulde G. Emergency medicine in modern Europe. *Emerg. Med. Australas.* 2007 Aug;19(4):300-2.

[122] Steinmetz J, Barnung S, Nielsen SL, Risom M, Rasmussen LS. Improved survival after an out-of-hospital cardiac arrest using new guidelines. *Acta Anaesthesiol. Scand.* 2008 Aug;52(7):908-13.

[123] Hallstrom AP, Cobb LA, Johnson E, Copass MK. Dispatcher assisted CPR: implementation and potential benefit. A 12-year study. *Resuscitation.* 2003 May;57(2):123-9.

[124] Rea TD, Eisenberg MS, Culley LL, Becker L. Dispatcher-assisted cardiopulmonary resuscitation and survival in cardiac arrest. *Circulation.* 2001 Nov 20;104(21):2513-6.

[125] Culley LL, Clark JJ, Eisenberg MS, Larsen MP. Dispatcher-assisted telephone CPR: common delays and time standards for delivery. *Ann. Emerg. Med.* 1991 Apr;20(4):362-6.

[126] Lecky F, Bryden D, Little R, Tong N, Moulton C. Emergency intubation for acutely ill and injured patients2009 Contract No.: 2.

[127] Iwami T, Nichol G, Hiraide A, Hayashi Y, Nishiuchi T, Kajino K, et al. Continuous improvements in "chain of survival" increased survival after out-of-hospital cardiac arrests: a large-scale population-based study. *Circulation.* 2009 Feb 10;119(5):728-34.

[128] Stiell IG, Wells GA, Field B, Spaite DW, Nesbitt LP, De Maio VJ, et al. Advanced cardiac life support in out-of-hospital cardiac arrest. *N. Engl. J. Med.* 2004 Aug 12;351(7):647-56.

[129] Rumball CJ, MacDonald D. The PTL, Combitube, laryngeal mask, and oral airway: a randomized prehospital comparative study of ventilatory device effectiveness and cost-effectiveness in 470 cases of cardiorespiratory arrest. *Prehosp. Emerg. Care.* 1997 Jan-Mar;1(1):1-10.

[130] ILCOR. Part 4: Advanced Life Support. Circulation. 2005 November 29;112(Suppl. 1):III-25 - III-54.

[131] Hubloue I, Lauwaert I, Corne L. Adrenaline dosage during cardiopulmonary resuscitation: a critical review. *Eur. J. Emerg. Med.* 1994 Sep;1(3):149-53.

[132] Marwick TH, Case C, Siskind V, Woodhouse SP. Adverse effect of early high-dose adrenaline on outcome of ventricular fibrillation. *Lancet.* 1988 Jul 9;2(8602):66-8.

[133] Goetting MG, Paradis NA. High-dose epinephrine improves outcome from pediatric cardiac arrest. *Ann. Emerg. Med.* 1991 Jan;20(1):22-6.

[134] Stiell IG, Hebert PC, Weitzman BN, Wells GA, Raman S, Stark RM, et al. High-dose epinephrine in adult cardiac arrest. *N. Engl. J. Med.* 1992 Oct 8;327(15):1045-50.

[135] Brown CG, Martin DR, Pepe PE, Stueven H, Cummins RO, Gonzalez E, et al. A comparison of standard-dose and high-dose epinephrine in cardiac arrest outside the hospital. The Multicenter High-Dose Epinephrine Study Group. *N. Engl. J .Med.* 1992 Oct 8;327(15):1051-5.

[136] Lipman J, Wilson W, Kobilski S, Scribante J, Lee C, Kraus P, et al. High-dose adrenaline in adult in-hospital asystolic cardiopulmonary resuscitation: a double-blind randomised trial. *Anaesth Intensive Care.* 1993 Apr;21(2):192-6.

[137] Carvolth RD, Hamilton AJ. Comparison of high-dose epinephrine versus standard-dose epinephrine in adult cardiac arrest in the prehospital setting. *Prehosp. Disaster Med.* 1996 Jul-Sep;11(3):219-22.

[138] Wyer PC, Perera P, Jin Z, Zhou Q, Cook DJ, Walter SD, et al. Vasopressin or epinephrine for out-of-hospital cardiac arrest. *Ann. Emerg. Med.* 2006 Jul;48(1):86-97.

[139] Little K, Auchincloss J, Reaves C. A mechanical cardiopulmonary life-support system. *Resuscitation.* 1974;3:63-8.

[140] Rozenberg A, Incagnoli P, Delpech P, Spaulding C, Vivien B, Kern KB, et al. Prehospital use of minimally invasive direct cardiac massage (MID-CM): a pilot study. *Resuscitation.* 2001 Sep;50(3):257-62.

[141] Kudenchuk PJ. Advanced cardiac life support antiarrhythmic drugs. *Cardiol. Clin.* 2002 Feb;20(1):79-87.

[142] Dorian P, Cass D, Schwartz B, Cooper R, Gelaznikas R, Barr A. Amiodarone as compared with lidocaine for shock-resistant ventricular fibrillation. *N. Engl. J. Med.* 2002 Mar 21;346(12):884-90.

[143] Lang E, Raisi M. Ventricular tachyarrhythmias (out of hospital cardiac arrests). *BMJ Clinical Evidence.* 2006;07(216):1-7.

[144] Marill KA, deSouza IS, Nishijima DK, Stair TO, Setnik GS, Ruskin JN. Amiodarone is poorly effective for the acute termination of ventricular tachycardia. *Ann. Emerg. Med.* 2006 Mar;47(3):217-24.

[145] Dell'Orfano JT, Naccarelli GV. Update on external cardioversion and defibrillation. *Curr.pin .Cardiol.* 2001 Jan;16(1):54-7.

[146] Faddy SC, Powell J, Craig JC. Biphasic and monophasic shocks for transthoracic defibrillation: a meta analysis of randomised controlled trials. *Resuscitation.* 2003 Jul;58(1):9-16.

[147] Reddy RK, Gleva MJ, Gliner BE, Dolack GL, Kudenchuk PJ, Poole JE, et al. Biphasic transthoracic defibrillation causes fewer ECG ST-segment changes after shock. *Ann. Emerg. Med.* 1997 Aug;30(2):127-34.

[148] Ambler JJ, Deakin CD. A randomized controlled trial of efficacy and ST change following use of the Welch-Allyn MRL PIC biphasic waveform versus damped sine monophasic waveform for external DC cardioversion. *Resuscitation.* 2006 Nov;71(2):146-51.

[149] Forcina MS, Farhat AY, O'Neil WW, Haines DE. Cardiac arrest survival after implementation of automated external defibrillator technology in the in-hospital setting. *Crit Care Med.* 2009 Apr;37(4):1229-36.

[150] Freeman K, Hendey GW, Shalit M, Stroh G. Biphasic defibrillation does not improve outcomes compared to monophasic defibrillation in out-of-hospital cardiac arrest. *Prehosp. Emerg. Care.* 2008 Apr-Jun;12(2):152-6.

[151] Bernard SA, Gray TW, Buist MD, Jones BM, Silvester W, Gutteridge G, et al. Treatment of comatose survivors of out-of-hospital cardiac arrest with induced hypothermia. *N. Engl. J. Med.* 2002 Feb 21;346(8):557-63.

[152] Mild therapeutic hypothermia to improve the neurologic outcome after cardiac arrest. *N. Engl. J. Med.* 2002 Feb 21;346(8):549-56.

[153] Guideline 11.9: Therapeutic Hypothermia After Cardiac Arrest: Australian Resuscitation Council2006.

[154] Vaillancourt C, Stiell IG, Wells GA. Understanding and improving low bystander CPR rates: a systematic review of the literature. *CJEM.* 2008 Jan;10(1):51-65.

[155] Bohm K, Rosenqvist M, Herlitz J, Hollenberg J, Svensson L. Survival is similar after standard treatment and chest compression only in out-of-hospital bystander cardiopulmonary resuscitation. *Circulation.* 2007 Dec 18;116(25):2908-12.

[156] Dias JA, Brown TB, Saini D, Shah RC, Cofield SS, Waterbor JW, et al. Simplified dispatch-assisted CPR instructions outperform standard protocol. *Resuscitation.* 2007 Jan;72(1):108-14.

[157] Chamberlain D. The International Liaison Committee on Resuscitation (ILCOR)-past and present: compiled by the Founding Members of the International Liaison Committee on Resuscitation. *Resuscitation.* 2005 Nov-Dec;67(2-3):157-61.

[158] Cummins RO, Chamberlain DA, Abramson NS, Allen M, Baskett PJ, Becker L, et al. Recommended guidelines for uniform reporting of data

from out-of-hospital cardiac arrest: the Utstein Style. A statement for health professionals from a task force of the American Heart Association, the European Resuscitation Council, the Heart and Stroke Foundation of Canada, and the Australian Resuscitation Council. *Circulation.* 1991 Aug;84(2):960-75.

[159] ILCOR. Part 1: Introduction. Circulation. 2005 November 29;112(Suppl. 1):III-1 - III-4.

[160] ILCOR. Part 2: Adult Basic Life Support. Circulation. 2005 November 29;112(Suppl. 1):III-5 - III-16.

[161] ILCOR. Part 3: Defibrillation. Circulation. 2005 November 29;112(Suppl. 1):III-17 - III-24.

[162] Jacobs IG, Morley P. New Changes to Resuscitation Guidelines2006 March 27.

[163] Hazinski MF, Nolan JP, Becker LB, Steen PA. Controversial Topics From the 2005 International Consensus Conference on Cardiopulmonary Resuscitation and Emergency Cardiovascular Care Science With Treatment Recommendations. *Circulation.* 2005 November 29;112(Suppl. 1):III-133 - III-6.

[164] Kerber RE, Martins JB, Kienzle MG, Constantin L, Olshansky B, Hopson R, et al. Energy, current, and success in defibrillation and cardioversion: clinical studies using an automated impedance-based method of energy adjustment. *Circulation.* 1988 May;77(5):1038-46.

[165] Weisfeldt ML, Becker LB. Resuscitation after cardiac arrest: a 3-phase time-sensitive model. *JAMA.* 2002 Dec 18;288(23):3035-8.

[166] Campbell RL, Hess EP, Atkinson EJ, White RD. Assessment of a three-phase model of out-of-hospital cardiac arrest in patients with ventricular fibrillation. *Resuscitation.* 2007 May;73(2):229-35.

[167] Gilmore CM, Rea TD, Becker LJ, Eisenberg MS. Three-phase model of cardiac arrest: time-dependent benefit of bystander cardiopulmonary resuscitation. *Am. J. Cardiol.* 2006 Aug 15;98(4):497-9.

[168] Vilke GM, Chan TC, Dunford JV, Metz M, Ochs G, Smith A, et al. The three-phase model of cardiac arrest as applied to ventricular fibrillation in a large, urban emergency medical services system. *Resuscitation.* 2005 Mar;64(3):341-6.

[169] Ornato JP, Gonzalez ER, Coyne MR, Beck CL, Collins MS. Arterial pH in out-of-hospital cardiac arrest: response time as a determinant of acidosis. *Am. J. Emerg. Med.* 1985 Nov;3(6):498-502.

[170] Idris AH, Becker LB, Fuerst RS, Wenzel V, Rush WJ, Melker RJ, et al. Effect of ventilation on resuscitation in an animal model of cardiac arrest. *Circulation.* 1994 Dec;90(6):3063-9.

[171] Kerber RE, Sarnat W. Factors influencing the success of ventricular defibrillation in man. *Circulation.* 1979 Aug;60(2):226-30.

[172] Eftestol T, Wik L, Sunde K, Steen PA. Effects of cardiopulmonary resuscitation on predictors of ventricular fibrillation defibrillation success during out-of-hospital cardiac arrest. *Circulation.* 2004 Jul 6;110(1):10-5.

[173] Reed MJ, Clegg GR, Robertson CE. Analysing the ventricular fibrillation waveform. *Resuscitation.* 2003 Apr;57(1):11-20.

[174] Menegazzi JJ, Callaway CW, Sherman LD, Hostler DP, Wang HE, Fertig KC, et al. Ventricular fibrillation scaling exponent can guide timing of defibrillation and other therapies. *Circulation.* 2004 Feb 24;109(7):926-31.

[175] A comparison of antiarrhythmic-drug therapy with implantable defibrillators in patients resuscitated from near-fatal ventricular arrhythmias. The Antiarrhythmics versus Implantable Defibrillators (AVID) Investigators. *N. Engl. J. Med.* 1997 Nov 27;337(22):1576-83.

[176] Connolly SJ, Gent M, Roberts RS, Dorian P, Roy D, Sheldon RS, et al. Canadian implantable defibrillator study (CIDS) : a randomized trial of the implantable cardioverter defibrillator against amiodarone. *Circulation.* 2000 Mar 21;101(11):1297-302.

[177] Connolly SJ, Hallstrom AP, Cappato R, Schron EB, Kuck KH, Zipes DP, et al. Meta-analysis of the implantable cardioverter defibrillator secondary prevention trials. AVID, CASH and CIDS studies. Antiarrhythmics vs Implantable Defibrillator study. Cardiac Arrest Study Hamburg . Canadian Implantable Defibrillator Study. *Eur .Heart. J.* 2000 Dec;21(24):2071-8.

[178] White RD, Blackwell TH, Russell JK, Snyder DE, Jorgenson DB. Transthoracic impedance does not affect defibrillation, resuscitation or survival in patients with out-of-hospital cardiac arrest treated with a non-escalating biphasic waveform defibrillator. *Resuscitation.* 2005 Jan;64(1):63-9.

[179] Garcia LA, Allan JJ, Kerber RE. Interactions between CPR and defibrillation waveforms: effect on resumption of a perfusing rhythm after defibrillation. *Resuscitation.* 2000 Nov;47(3):301-5.

[180] Niemann JT, Cairns CB, Sharma J, Lewis RJ. Treatment of prolonged ventricular fibrillation. Immediate countershock versus high-dose epinephrine and CPR preceding countershock. *Circulation.* 1992 Jan;85(1):281-7.

[181] Niemann JT, Cruz B, Garner D, Lewis RJ. Immediate countershock versus cardiopulmonary resuscitation before countershock in a 5-minute swine model of ventricular fibrillation arrest. *Ann. Emerg. Med.* 2000 Dec;36(6):543-6.

[182] Yakaitis RW, Ewy GA, Otto CW, Taren DL, Moon TE. Influence of time and therapy on ventricular defibrillation in dogs. *Crit. Care Med.* 1980 Mar;8(3):157-63.

[183] Menegazzi JJ, Davis EA, Yealy DM, Molner RL, Nicklas KA, Hosack GM, et al. An experimental algorithm versus standard advanced cardiac life support in a swine model of out-of-hospital cardiac arrest. *Ann. Emerg. Med.* 1993 Feb;22(2):235-9.

[184] Menegazzi JJ, Seaberg DC, Yealy DM, Davis EA, MacLeod BA. Combination pharmacotherapy with delayed countershock vs standard advanced cardiac life support after prolonged ventricular fibrillation. *Prehosp. Emerg. Care.* 2000 Jan-Mar;4(1):31-7.

[185] Niemann JT, Rosborough JP, Youngquist S, Thomas J, Lewis RJ. Is all ventricular fibrillation the same? A comparison of ischemically induced with electrically induced ventricular fibrillation in a porcine cardiac arrest and resuscitation model. *Crit. Care Med.* 2007 May;35(5):1356-61.

[186] Pepe PE, Fowler RL, Roppolo LP, Wigginton JG. Clinical review: Reappraising the concept of immediate defibrillatory attempts for out-of-hospital ventricular fibrillation. *Crit. Care.* 2004 Feb;8(1):41-5.

[187] Hallstrom AP, Ornato JP, Weisfeldt M, Travers A, Christenson J, McBurnie MA, et al. Public-access defibrillation and survival after out-of-hospital cardiac arrest. *N. Engl. J. Med.* 2004 Aug 12;351(7):637-46.

[188] Weaver WD, Cobb LA, Hallstrom AP, Fahrenbruch C, Copass MK, Ray R. Factors influencing survival after out-of-hospital cardiac arrest. *J. Am. Coll. Cardiol.* 1986 Apr;7(4):752-7.

[189] Valenzuela TD, Spaite DW, Meislin HW, Clark LL, Wright AL, Ewy GA. Emergency vehicle intervals versus collapse-to-CPR and collapse-to-defibrillation intervals: monitoring emergency medical services system performance in sudden cardiac arrest. *Ann. Emerg. Med.* 1993 Nov;22(11):1678-83.

[190] Martens P, Vandekerckhove Y. Optimal defibrillation strategy and follow-up of out-of-hospital cardiac arrest. The Belgian CPCR Study Group. *Resuscitation.* 1996 Feb;31(1):25-32.

[191] Ladwig KH, Schoefinius A, Danner R, Gurtler R, Herman R, Koeppel A, et al. Effects of early defibrillation by ambulance personnel on short- and

long-term outcome of cardiac arrest survival: the Munich experiment. *Chest.* 1997 Dec;112(6):1584-91.

[192] Kern KB, Garewal HS, Sanders AB, Janas W, Nelson J, Sloan D, et al. Depletion of myocardial adenosine triphosphate during prolonged untreated ventricular fibrillation: effect on defibrillation success. *Resuscitation.* 1990 Dec;20(3):221-9.

[193] Ditchey RV, Horwitz LD. Metabolic evidence of inadequate coronary blood flow during closed-chest resuscitation in dogs. *Cardiovasc Res.* 1985 Jul;19(7):419-25.

[194] Grover FL, Fewel JG, Ghidoni JJ, Norton JB, Arom KV, Trinkle JK. Effects of ventricular fibrillation on coronary blood flow and myocardial metabolism. *J. Thorac. Cardiovasc. Surg.* 1977 Apr;73(4):616-24.

[195] Babbs CF. Circulatory adjuncts. Newer methods of cardiopulmonary resuscitation. *Cardiol. Clin.* 2002 Feb;20(1):37-59.

[196] Weil MH, Tang W. Cardiopulmonary resuscitation: a promise as yet largely unfulfilled. *Dis. Mon.* 1997 Jul;43(7):429-501.

[197] Walcott GP, Killingsworth CR, Ideker RE. Do clinically relevant transthoracic defibrillation energies cause myocardial damage and dysfunction? *Resuscitation.* 2003 Oct;59(1):59-70.

[198] Cummins RO, Ornato JP, Thies WH, Pepe PE. Improving survival from sudden cardiac arrest: the "chain of survival" concept. A statement for health professionals from the Advanced Cardiac Life Support Subcommittee and the Emergency Cardiac Care Committee, American Heart Association. *Circulation.* 1991 May;83(5):1832-47.

[199] Stiell IG, Wells GA, Field BJ, Spaite DW, De Maio VJ, Ward R, et al. Improved out-of-hospital cardiac arrest survival through the inexpensive optimization of an existing defibrillation program: OPALS study phase II. Ontario Prehospital Advanced Life Support. *JAMA.* 1999 Apr 7;281(13):1175-81.

[200] Vaillancourt C, Lui A, De Maio VJ, Wells GA, Stiell IG. Socioeconomic status influences bystander CPR and survival rates for out-of-hospital cardiac arrest victims. *Resuscitation.* 2008 Dec;79(3):417-23.

[201] Stecher FS, Olsen JA, Stickney RE, Wik L. Transthoracic impedance used to evaluate performance of cardiopulmonary resuscitation during out of hospital cardiac arrest. *Resuscitation.* 2008 Dec;79(3):432-7.

[202] Skogvoll E, Nordseth T. The early minutes of in-hospital cardiac arrest: Shock or CPR? A population based prospective study. *Scand J. Trauma Resusc. Emerg. Med.* 2008;16(1):11.

[203] Peberdy MA, Kaye W, Ornato JP, Larkin GL, Nadkarni V, Mancini ME, et al. Cardiopulmonary resuscitation of adults in the hospital: a report of 14720 cardiac arrests from the National Registry of Cardiopulmonary Resuscitation. *Resuscitation.* 2003 Sep;58(3):297-308.

INDEX